JUMP OFF
THE DIET
TREADMILL

12 Weeks on Your Way
to Lifetime Weight Loss

TZABIA SIEGEL

True Health Publications, 53 Dingwall Avenue, Toronto, Ontario, M4J 1C4

The information contained in this book is intended to provide supportive and educational material on the subject covered. It is not intended to serve as a replacement for medical or nutritional advice from a professional. The author and publisher expressly disclaim any liability, loss, or risk, personal or otherwise, which is incurred as a consequence, direct or indirect, of the use or application of the contents of this book.

National Library of Canada Cataloguing in Publication

Siegel, Tzabia
    Jump Off the Diet Treadmill: 12 Weeks on Your Way to Lifetime Weight Loss
    / Tzabia Siegel

Includes bibliographical references and index.
ISBN 978-0-9918272-0-6

Book design by Jera Publishing
Book cover design by Jun Ares, Mark Siegel and Jera Publishing

This book is dedicated to all my individual and group clients, past and present, who with their open minds and willing actions, have inspired me to learn more, and become better at what I do. Thank you for giving back to me as much as you have received.

And to Barry, for providing me with the foundation of love, support, and security that has allowed me to get on with my work. You really are my beaver.

Contents

JUMP OFF
THE DIET
TREADMILL

*12 Weeks on Your Way
to Lifetime Weight Loss*

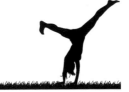

Introduction

Meet three of my clients.

First, Jeannie. Mid-thirties, creative professional, has traveled extensively, highly intelligent and a critical thinker. Jeannie grew up in a strict religious family where meals were somber events, which included finishing everything on her plate whether she was hungry or not. She obsesses about food and doesn't feel at ease in her body.

Barb is fifty-one, married, with two kids in university. After years as a stay-at-home mom, she went back to work as a legal secretary. Her kids, husband, work and community have been her priorities over the years. Because of this, there has been little time to take care of her self. She has gained weight progressively, doesn't feel sexy, and is ready for change.

Charles is a successful entrepreneur/consultant. He was an athlete in college and remains active but has developed a gut that so many men get as they age. He remembers what it was like to be in great shape and knows that with the right support, he can turn his achievement-oriented nature to his advantage.

Each client shares the common ground that they want to lose weight and be healthy – and they have come to me because they know that diets don't work. They need guidance to find out what does. Between the three of them they have tried all of the major dieting programs, which included a doctor who performed injections and deprived them of calories, tracking points online, buying programmed meals, expensive detoxes, and various forms of fasting. Each person has lost weight a number of times, but not one of them was able to sustain it.

I can relate. My own attempts to control my eating were met with only temporary success until I figured out that I was missing the big picture. The big picture is a connection to our humanity – that complex need that we have for comfort, soulfulness, purpose, simplicity, balance, outlets of expression, excitement, safety – essentially the mix of body, mind and soul. Without the connection to what makes us human, we get temporary solutions and long-term failure. Our inability to lose weight and keep it off is then perceived as a weakness: of will, of self-control, of commitment. The reality however, is that it is rarely a character issue. Rather it is a need to clarify and refocus our energies in ways that address the underlying causes of being heavy.

Jump off the Diet Treadmill takes you on a journey into both your physiology and your behavior. It has been born out of the experiences of hundreds of clients, people like you, who have successfully stepped off the treadmill and found it to be far easier than they thought to break the cycle of on-again, off-again dieting. This book is intended to serve as a practical and insightful guidebook, balanced between the science of nutrition and the art of nourishment.

It is designed with your fast-paced (potentially overwhelming) life in mind. It assumes that you are intelligent but very busy, and so it attempts to make each step simple, doable and understandable. But it also encourages you to stretch beyond your comfort zone in order to reach higher and more sustainable goals.

The book begins with an explanation of the principles that underlie the program. Following the principles, each week includes one aspect that will affect your physiology directly (food, movement, rest) and one aspect of behavior (mind, emotion, soul) that builds the foundation for long-term success. We move step-by-step through the 12-weeks, framing each week with education and insight that explains:

- What you need to do.
- Why you need to do it.
- How you can do it.

The weeks have been organized in an order that builds the foundation first and then adds to that foundation. If I had my choice, everyone would start at the beginning and then move progressively through the weeks. However, there's a wide range of needs. Follow your instincts. For you, the greatest value may come from the insights on sustainable eating; or it may be from a deeper understanding of your behavior or from a combination of both. If you do skip around, I encourage you to also check back with what you have missed to make sure you have that component in place. If it takes you longer than twelve weeks to develop all the practices that work for you, then be patient. Relax into it. You have your whole life ahead of you.

A last note: There is nothing that I ask my clients to do or that I suggest in this book that I haven't done myself. During the mid-eighties, in three months, I lost the extra twenty pounds that I had carried since my early teens using what is laid out in this book. I have sustained my ideal weight by weaving the tools and techniques that are most powerful for me into my daily life.

With an open mind, a willingness to take action and a patient mindset, I trust that you will find the practices that work most powerfully for you. Have fun. Enjoy the journey.

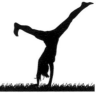

The Underlying Principles of *Jump Off the Diet Treadmill*

1. Change is possible

When you have tried many times to achieve something as challenging as long term weight loss and have not been successful, you identify with that failure. One more program, book, or self-proclaimed expert has you hoping -- but not necessarily believing -- that it is possible to be healthy and light for the rest of your life. *Jump Off the Diet Treadmill* can't promise anything more than what you are ready for. However it offers the possibility for real change if are open to new perspectives and willing to take action, likely in a different way than you have done previously. I have seen how change is not only possible, but is *probable* when a person is ready to get their mind and soul on board with their body.

2. Get to know your brain

There is nothing like a little neuroscience to help you understand why you do what you do. What you think is a flaw in your character (a lack of will-power as an example) is put into perspective when you know more about how your brain works. To that end, you'll find examples of the brain's functioning peppered throughout the book. Neuroscience is a complex topic and in no way do I proclaim to be an expert in any facet of it. However even a little brain knowledge can take you a long way towards understanding an important element of what drives your behavior. I find it fascinating, and as I have shared what I've learned with my clients, they have consistently claimed it to be useful to release themselves from self-judgment.

3. Commit to health as your first priority

Steady energy throughout the day, clear thinking, stable emotions, being free of pain and discomfort are signs of good health. Losing weight and keeping it off is dependent on the strength of these qualities. You'll need energy, clarity, and focused planning to support your efforts to eat well, to exercise and to embark on other nourishing activities. Pain and sickness will hold you back and slow you down. Focusing on your health is a shift in perspective from judgment about your weight to caring for your body.

4. Sustainability is the name of the game

Ninety-five percent of people who go on a diet will regain the weight that they have lost within one to five years. I'm not interested in you being part of that statistic. The mission of this book is to guide you towards a way of eating, and relating to food and your body, that you can practice for the rest of your life. Keep in mind however, that sustainable weight loss isn't just about being thinner. It's about living differently, about living a part of yourself that has yet to be fulfilled. You are taking a new path. This requires more than just desire. The requirements are to be open-minded, willing and persistent. Commitment will be rewarded with not only a loss of weight, but also a sense that you are finally in control of this part of your life.

5. Take it one step at a time

Few people have the time or resources to make big change quickly and in a way that they can sustain. Besides, taking on big change too quickly will trigger survival mechanisms in your brain that will sabotage your efforts. Think of the diets that you have been on, trying to eliminate the 'bad' foods and add in the 'good' foods all at once. Did they work in the long run? I'm guessing you wouldn't be here if they did. Lasting change is about making a commitment to taking on only one, or maybe two new things each week, which you can repeat over and over again until it becomes second nature.

6. Check your expectations at the door

Let's face it. We do not live in a culture that promotes patience. On the contrary, we are surrounded by instant gratification with thousands of promises made about losing weight fast, and endless options for fast convenient food. In the midst of this, you have developed habits that will take time to break down and replace with healthier habits. It may not happen as fast as you want. So relax. Check in on your goals to see if they are realistic relative to everything else that's happening in your life. Consider the amount of time that you have, your starting point, your history, your present health and your energy level, before you determine what's doable. Set yourself up for success by being realistic rather than priming yourself for failure by expecting too much in too short a period of time. By being realistic about the expectations that you have for yourself, you are more likely to continue to move forward rather than fall off the wagon and stay off -- which brings us to our next principle.

7. Fall off the wagon? Get back on as soon as you can

This is one of the keys that will make the long haul doable. Let go of your all-or-nothing, "I just blew my diet, I might as well eat everything I can get my hands on" attitude. Indulge a little. Have some fun. And then forgive yourself and get on with it. Don't waste energy beating yourself up. You ate one meal that's not ideal? Oh well. Next meal, get back on track. Two or three meals, not ideal? Ok, breathe. No better time than now to jump back on that wagon. You can do it at anytime and at any meal. If you've ever wondered how that co-worker, neighbor or relative manages to maintain their weight despite their indulgences, you can guarantee that they have this figured out. It is an imperative to sustainability because food is one of life's great pleasures. If you believe for one minute that you can maintain a restrictive diet for the rest of your life, wake up and taste the reality of homemade ice cream. This is about creating a balance between healthy choices and sweet or salty indulgence. Pleasure is part of the joy of being human. You don't want to miss out on it. But you also need to be able to handle it without losing control. Freedom comes with deeper self-aware-ness, conscious moderation and choosing quality over quantity. And it starts with getting back on the wagon that you just fell off of.

8. We get good at whatever we practice

Think of the thoughts, feelings and actions that are habitual for you. You have practiced these over and over again so that you have created well-en-trenched pathways between your brain and the rest of your body. These 'neural pathways' make it easy for you to repeat those thoughts, feelings and actions because through practice you have made them automatic. This book will ask you to take on new perspectives and skills. As you create changes and repeat them over time, they will become easier and easier to do. This concept of practice is not difficult to grasp when you think about learning new physical skills, such as riding a bike or getting down the rou-tines in a fitness class. But it is equally applicable to the thoughts that you run and the emotions that you get caught up in repeatedly. They are as powerful as your actions (some would argue more so) because they exert control over your physiology, affecting your metabolism as well as driv-ing you towards your behavior. In *Jump off the Diet Treadmill*, you will be guided to pay attention to not only what you eat and the quality of your exercise and rest, but also to how you think and feel about your body and yourself. Practice what you wish to become.

Week #1

· · · · · · · · · · · · · ·

Make Friends with Protein

· · ·

Find Your Motivation

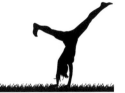

Make Friends with Protein

What You Need To Do

Considering friendship as a desire to hang out with someone, to confide in, to be endeared to – I am using the concept of befriending liberally here. The point is that I am inviting you to get to know protein more intimately. If I told you now that you need to eat protein at every meal, it would be too much to take on all at once. That is, however, what you're aiming for. For now, take your time getting to know which proteins you like, which options make the most sense for each meal, approximately how much and why you need to eat them. Then one meal at a time, start adding them in. If you are already eating protein at some meals, that's great. Now you can work on increasing the portion, improving the quality, and varying the types.

Why You Need To Do It

Our bodies are these amazing cell production factories – every day somewhere in the range of three hundred billion new cells are replaced, repaired and regenerated. Phenomenal stuff. Proteins offer the building blocks to these billions of cells. Tissues, enzymes, some brain chemicals and some hormones rely on the amino acids in protein to provide the structure upon which they are built. For the sake of weight loss, protein is the hero in numerous ways. Here are three to consider:

1. The presence of protein stimulates the fat burning hormone, GLUCAGON

Eating too many carbs leads to those carbs being stored as sugar in the muscles and liver. (We'll talk more about this later). If there is excess sugar beyond what can be stored in those tissues, the extra supply makes its way to the fat cells where it is formed into fat/sugar molecules. Glucagon is the hormone that stimulates the fat/sugar molecules stored in the fat cells, to be transported from those cells so they can be burned for energy. If you want to shrink your fat cells, you need glucagon, which is released when you eat protein.

2. Eating protein helps to stabilize your blood sugar and reduces cravings

Glucagon also plays a role in ensuring that there is a balanced supply of sugar as a fuel source for the brain, muscles and tissues. If the supply of carbs/sugar is erratic, you will experience any number of symptoms that will make it difficult to maintain your energy and focus and will lead to cravings and binge eating. Symptoms of blood sugar irregularity are apparent when you go too long without eating a balanced meal with protein, and include the following:

- Headaches
- Low energy, fatigue
- Dizziness, faintness or light-headedness
- Irritability
- Nervousness or anxiousness
- Calmer after eating
- Sporadic 'highs' and 'lows' throughout the day
- Crave a lift from carbohydrates, sugar or alcohol, and then experience a drop in energy after eating them
- Frequent urination
- Frequent thirst
- Difficulty staying asleep

3. Protein stabilizes your mood, helps you focus and reduces cravings in another way

Our brains are programmed for pleasure. We want satisfaction and comfort. To have it we need an abundance of the pleasure and satiation related brain chemicals. Guess how they're made? Protein. Yup. Surprise! The amino acids that are the building blocks of protein provide the raw material for the pleasure and satiation hormones dopamine, serotonin, leptin, CCK. With those hormones in balance, you will find that the need to seek comfort through sugar, fat and salt is lessened. With the physical cravings minimized – you will have more resources to deal with the psychological cravings.

I can't emphasize the importance of protein enough. I have seen reductions in clients' cravings, more energy, focus and stable moods within days when they eat enough protein consistently throughout the day.

How You Can Do It

The first thing you need to do is be clear on what constitutes protein. You probably already know this, but in case you need a refresher or want to double check, here is a list of proteins. I would suggest that you check off the ones that you like.

FISH	whitefish, salmon, tuna, mackerel, sardines, trout, plus others
SEAFOOD	shrimp, prawns, scallops, mussels, clams, lobster, crab
EGGS	preferably pasture raised, organic or at least free range
POULTRY	chicken, turkey, duck, pheasant, any other bird
MEATS	venison, beef, lamb, buffalo, pork, goat, any other mammal
DAIRY	cottage cheese, ricotta cheese, yogurt (particularly Greek style), cheese

PROTEIN POWDERS	whey, vegan sources from sprouted grains and beans, fermented soy
SOY	edamame, tofu, tempeh, miso, natto
LEGUMES	black beans, kidney beans, lentils, chickpeas, plus others *
GRAINS	amaranth, buckwheat, barley, oats, wild and colored rice, quinoa, millet, plus others *
NUTS AND SEEDS	almonds, Brazil nuts, walnuts, pumpkin, sunflower, sesame, plus others

How many servings of protein do you need to eat?

Although you are just getting to be friends with protein this week, you will eventually be working towards eating some protein in combination with some other foods (more on that coming up in the following weeks) every three to four hours throughout the day. That means that you will be working towards four to six servings of protein every day. Let's use five meals as the average for most people. Five meals per day equals thirty-five per week. That's the overall number of servings. Now you can break it down to determine how many servings of each source of protein you are going to aim for in each week.

Step 1   List the proteins that you like and would be willing to eat on a weekly basis.

Step 2   Note the usual number of servings for each of those proteins that you presently eat in a week.

Step 3   Now add up the total to see how many servings you are presently getting.

Step 4   Subtract the number of servings that you are presently getting from your weekly protein goal. (Goals are 28 if you are eating 4 meals per day, 35 if you are eating 5 meals, 42 if you are eating 6 meals).

Don't get discouraged if it seems that you are far off your mark. Remember this is a one-step-at-a-time process. For now, you are just working on figuring out what you need to do. Then you will start to take action on it.

Step **5** Note how many of each of your preferred proteins you think you would be able to commit to in a week to get to your goal number.

* *

For example, my client Jeannie that I introduced you to loves chicken, cottage cheese, salmon, and Greek yogurt. She was also eating chickpeas, beef, eggs and other cheeses one or two times per week. This was her approximate protein intake when she started:

Chicken	4X	Beef	1X
Cottage Cheese	4X	Eggs	2X
Salmon	1X	Other cheese	2X
Greek yogurt	6X	Total protein servings per week	20

In figuring out what she was willing to eat to get her protein servings up to the needed amount, here is what she came up with:

Chicken	4X	Eggs	3X
Cottage Cheese	4X	Beans	2X
Salmon or another fish/seafood	4X	Whey protein shake	5X
Greek yogurt	6X	Other cheese	2X
Beef	1X	Nuts and seeds	3X

Now her total servings of protein per week are equal to 34. She did this by adding in more fish, eggs, nuts and seeds, beans and a protein shake once per day, 5 days per week. Did she do this all at once? Absolutely not. It took her about six weeks to get to the point where she was eating enough protein, five out of seven days in the week. The other two days (on the weekend) she wanted to stay more flexible for her social life. Even then however, understanding the concept of choosing protein at every meal helped *her keep on track more often than not.*

* *

How much protein do you need in each serving?

This is a good question and not an easy one to answer.

No one can pinpoint exactly how much protein is needed because each person is biochemically unique, and their nutrient needs will vary. However, most people who need to lose weight would benefit from an increase, and sometimes a substantial increase in protein. My experience has been that when people increase their protein at every meal and snack, weight loss happens more readily.

Here is the general guideline. Aim for 20 – 40 grams of protein at each meal. I know that is a fairly wide range. The practical reality is that at some meals, particularly lunch and dinner, it will be easier to hit the higher range. At breakfast and snacks, you may find yourself within the lower range. Consult the chart on the following page to get a sense of the protein content of some foods.

Protein Content (in grams)

Seafood (6 oz)		Meat/Fowl (4 oz boneless)		Dairy (1 oz or 1 cup)		Beans and Grains (1/2c)	
clams, 9 large	23	beef, ground lean	20	cottage ch, 1 c	28	adzuki	9
cod	30	beef, round steak	22	ricotta, 1 c	28	black beans	7.5
crab	31	beef, sirloin	20	feta	4	chickpeas	7.5
haddock	32	beef, short ribs	16	hard cheeses	6-8	kidney beans	7
halibut	35	beef, tenderloin	21	cream cheese	2	lentils	8
lobster	32	lamb, chops w bone	16	goat, hard	9	soybeans	15
mackerel	32	lamb, leg w bone	17	goat, soft	5	tempeh, 4 oz	22
oysters, 6	6	pork, Cdn bacon	23	milk, 1 – 4% fat	8	tofu	10
pike	33	pork, ham	20	buttermilk	8	miso, 2 tb	4
salmon	34	pork, 1 chop, 6 oz	22	eggnog	10	rice, brown	3
sardines, 2	6	pork, spareribs	12	goat milk	9	rice, wild	4
scallops	27	veal, cutlet	18	sheep milk	15	quinoa	4
sea bass	30	veal, rib roast	16	soy milk	7	buckwheat	4
shrimp	35	chicken, breast	23	rice milk	1	barley	2
snapper	35	chicken, leg	20	almond milk	1	oats, whole	4
sole	32	chicken, wing	21	whey protein	24	wheat flour, wh	8
trout	36	turkey, light meat	24	yogurt, whole	8	rye flour, dark	10
tuna, 1/2 can	21	turkey, dark meat	22	yogurt, low fat	12	rye flour, light	4
whitefish	32	egg, 1 large	6	yogurt, no fat	13	cornmeal, wh	5
Nuts and Seeds							
Almonds, 16	4	Pecans, 8 halves	2	Pumpkin seed, 2tb	7	Sunflower sd, 2 tb	5

Figures sourced from: Nutrition Almanac, 5th Edition
by Lavon J. Dunne and www.nutritiondata.com

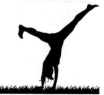

Find your Motivation

What you need to do

One of the biggest mistakes people make when they go on diets is that they try to get their body on board without the support of their mind. The body can't do this job alone. My experience with those who have been successful with the weight loss journey is that they have already created a lighter person in their own mind and they are patiently waiting for their body to catch up. And catch up it does. There is no one more powerful than a person who has 'made up his or her mind' and who knows 'that nothing, and no one, is going to veer them off that course'.

When I work one-on-one with clients, I prepare them for the challenges that lay ahead by describing the 'honeymoon period'. It's that time at the beginning, where everything is hopeful, exciting and new. Everyone is charged by the idea of finally tackling this weight loss issue forever. It's a lovely thought. Being in charge of your choices, having a great relationship with food, unburdening your mind. But along with the hope, I offer them a reality check. Even with the support that they're getting, they will hit the bumpy road of their old behaviors. It will take anywhere from two to six weeks until the patterns that they've been repeating for years, show up and push them off the wagon. It's likely to happen to you too. At that point, you might fall off the wagon and stay off. It's easy to go back to what you were doing before because, well, it's easy. The brain loves what it knows. It loves repetition and following well-entrenched patterns. It is only a strong motivational force that will make the difference between jumping back on or letting the wagon roll down the road and out of site.

Knowing what motivates you, whether it is positive or negative, or a little of each, is one of the first keys to getting back on that wagon when the road gets bumpy. Take your time reading the rest of this week's notes, considering your deepest motivations. Then start your practice of being in the place that makes you powerful.

Why you need to do it

Staying the course for the rest of your life relies on a deep emotional connection to why you are doing what you're doing. This deep connection is linked to what we would call 'internal motivation'. In the brain, internal motivation is a complex process where, in split seconds and unconsciously, you weigh out the strength of feelings for or against something and make a decision whether or not you should take action and what action you should take. This is happening without you being aware of it. It is driven by decisions and experiences you've had, and beliefs and perspectives that are already ingrained. Internal motivation is woven into who you are.

Compare that to 'external motivation'. Here, you make decisions that are deliberate and conscious. You are aware of what you are deciding. For example, most of us can relate to the resolution, made at the beginning of the new year, to go on a diet. You're going on a beach vacation in March and your goal is to lose twenty pounds so that you'll look good in a bathing suit. This is a reasonable desire (who doesn't want to look good in a bathing suit?). But if you have made that resolution multiple times without much effect, it's probably not synching with your much more powerful internal motivators. In fact, if your external motivation (like, looking good in a bikini) doesn't line up with your internal motivations (as an example, 'feeling calm' – potato chips give you the temporary feeling of calmness) you are ripe for discontent.

In coaching, we call our internal motivators 'values' and the well-known coaching line, at least amongst coaches, is that 'a fulfilled life is a life lived in alignment with our values'. In other words if we connect externally with what motivates us internally and act on it, we are on the path to a happy life.

Strong motivation is tied to and reflected by powerful emotions. You should be able to feel the juice running through you when you think about your goals and why you're doing them.

A client named Judy likened the challenge of conquering her food and weight issues as "Mount Everest beckoning me." She related to the mountain climber who is ready to take on her greatest challenge. Judy is driven by self-development. It is such a powerful value that seeing herself as the climber had a lot of emotional juice for her. She consciously used that charge to propel her through the challenging times on her route to losing forty-three pounds.

If you are aware of what is driving you to lose weight from the inside, you are more likely going to move towards vegetables and away from donuts, you will book time in your schedule to exercise and you will make a decision before you get to the party to keep the gluttony in check. On the other hand, without the strong emotions that are wrapped around powerful internal motivators, it will be easy to fall into the habits that are well known to you, but keep you weighed down.

I have talked to many people who were motivated to lose weight because of a personal health scare, or the death of a friend or family member. You probably know people like this. They were hit hard by their mortality and experienced the fear of impaired health or their impending death. For some, a strong emotion such as fear is so powerful as an internal motivator that it can catalyse long-term change. Interestingly, it has been mostly men that I have encountered who were motivated to make big change by this kind of fear. That has something to do with how their brains' function compared to women's. Men's brains register a threat with strong emotion and detailed memory much more so than a positive emotion. Women's brains, on the other hand, have complex circuitry to register all types of emotions, pleasant or unpleasant with greater detail and to store it in memory.

Either way, success at long-term weight loss demands that you tap into what's at the heart of your desire to change. Without a strong motivational force, it will be hard to stick with the process when it is so much easier to fall back into step with old habits that you know so well (and keep you heavy). Motivation is like a foundation that you build a house on. It's the structure that you build a healthy mind from which you can then create a healthy body.

Georgia is a woman in her mid-thirties who wanted to lose weight and develop a healthy relationship with food. She has a young daughter and one of her deepest motivators is the health and wellbeing of her child. Wanting to be a good role model became a powerful force for Georgia. She used her emotional connection to her daughter as the dangling carrot when she felt challenged in her self-care choices. A quick sensory image of playing and running with her daughter had enough emotional juice that it was a force for her decision-making. She felt that it was one of the key tools that got her on track to lose twenty-five pounds and to still maintain it four years later.

External motivation alone is not powerful enough to keep you on the wagon, if it is not in alignment with your internal motivators. External motivators tend to be verbal. (I am going to lose twenty pounds by March 15th) and are a response to a person's judgments and decisions (I should be twenty pounds lighter). They're often at the heart of temporary New Year's resolutions. They seem powerful at the time but soon fall by the wayside if they aren't supported by a deeper drive. That comes from the internal motivators. These are non-verbal and sensory-based (the feeling of being light and carefree) and tend to be based on an internal set of values (being a powerful contributor to your child's happiness).

The most compelling idea to note about internal and external motivation is that you can strengthen your drive by aligning them together. Identifying your external motivation and then using your imagination to experience those goals sensually (see, feel, hear the outcome that you want) is a well-used technique by sports psychologists and athletes and is available to us all. In addition, clarifying your internal motivators, stating them and writing them down, brings them into conscious awareness, providing you with strong focus.

Here rests the power to motivate – it is in your capacity to use your mind to identify what drives you and to imagine yourself as though you're already there. The brain interprets your sensory imagination as though it were reality so imagining your outcomes (positive or negative) supports you to make it real. It's the 'fake it 'til you make it' premise. Fake it or not, there is a biology to this premise, because each time you engage the senses with your imagination, the electrical and hormonal signals that are relayed throughout the body are the same as those that are sent out when it's actually happening. It is your imagination that will spark the connection between your internal and external motivation and will serve you well when you are taking on the challenge of breaking free of your habitual eating patterns.

How you can do it

There is a powerful basic need behind human motivation. It is the movement towards pleasure or away from pain. Since motivation is at the heart of the behaviours that drive us toward our goals, we can use both pleasure and pain to help you find and strengthen your commitment over the long-term.

Pleasure is where we begin.

Make a list. Consider it a kind of bucket list of the outcomes that you get from being light and healthy.

What are the positive outcomes of being healthy and at your ideal weight?

(I would suggest that you write them down).

Now, let's take it a step further. Consider what you value most in life. Is it family, connection, peace, achievement, fun, beauty, self-development, exploration, creativity, spirituality, nature, security?

If you were to list your top ten values, what would they be?

One way to think about this is in the form of another question.

What gives the most positive emotional feedback?

I have included a list of values below to spark your thoughts. Check off the ten that you consider most crucial to having a sense of fulfilment in your life.

☐ love	☐ joy	☐ health
☐ connection	☐ humour	☐ vitality
☐ intimacy	☐ fun	☐ balance
☐ belonging	☐ playfulness	☐ calm
☐ safety		
☐ security	☐ peace	☐ being of service
	☐ spirituality	☐ contribution
☐ beauty	☐ nature	☐ leadership
☐ sensuality	☐ oneness	☐ responsibility
☐ attractiveness	☐ humility	
☐ aesthetics		☐ being powerful
	☐ self-expression	☐ recognition
☐ adventure	☐ passion	☐ achievement
☐ freedom	☐ creativity	☐ influence
☐ risk-taking	☐ freedom	☐ excellence
☐ exploration	☐ independence	
☐ discovery	☐ uniqueness	☐ compassion
		☐ caring
☐ wisdom	☐ integrity	☐ kindness
☐ growth	☐ truth	☐ respect
☐ self-development	☐ honesty	☐ tolerance
☐ learning	☐ courage	☐ diversity
	☐ trustworthiness	☐ justice
☐ knowledge	☐ authenticity	
☐ intelligence		☐ order
☐ education		☐ organization

Thinking about your top ten values, what other positive outcomes (of reaching your goals for your body) can you throw into your bucket?

Once you have your list, move on to the next step.

You will need to be able to see it, feel it and sense these outcomes as a possibility. Without the sensations, it won't have an emotional charge for you. It has to have an emotional charge to be effective.

Imagine yourself as a thinner person. Direct your mind to any experience of being lighter using your senses of sight, sound and touch. Imagine seeing your reflection in a store window and loving what you see, take pleasure in the vision, look at the clothes you are wearing, see yourself walking, running, doing other activities, let your mind wander through the visual gratification. Test yourself in the imagination of sound, hearing the tone of your lighter voice, your laughter, hear yourself speaking to someone else telling them about your weight loss. Now get into the sensation of feeling, of walking briskly on a crisp fall day, taking those stairs two at a time, playing games with your children or grandchildren, feel yourself doing yoga or swimming. Let your imagination take you where you are most motivated to go. Use your bucket list of outcomes as a guideline to direct your attention.

Using your bucket list of outcomes will guide you to be specific with your imagination. You need to include the people, places and activities that matter most to you.

Imagine yourself at the finish line of the Boston marathon, playing a Mozart piano sonata, kicking the soccer ball with your son or daughter, laying on the beach in your itsy-bitsy bikini, leading a crowd in a political rally, wearing that favourite dress that you bought when you were first married or whatever else inspires you.

Let yourself dream.

How great would it be to feel more like yourself – to have the outside image match the inside you?

Write down a few details about what has the most emotional charge for you.

For example, it might be seeing yourself in the sun on the beach or feeling heat on your near-naked body or the sound of your own laughter. Get a clear sense of what this is for you so that you can return easily to it. For reference, I'll call this your 'place of pleasure.' However, you can identify it by giving it a name that is more personal to you. A client called his place 'The Beach.' Another named hers 'Free and Easy.'

Imagine your 'place of pleasure' at least five times per day over the next week so it gets well scorched into your mind.

Now let's move on to pain as a source of motivation.

The reality is that some people need to have their doctor remind them that they are likely to face the certainty of a heart attack like their father had, or get to the point of not being able to walk up a flight of stairs because they run out of breath in order to find any reason to change. If you need to wait for that, so be it. But wouldn't you prefer to deepen your motivation before you're staring death in the face or can barely walk anymore? Imagine you're already there so that you can get going on this before its too late.

. . . .

Think about not being with your kids or grandkids as they grow. Think about the pain that you are going to experience when your joints don't work anymore, or the shame of seeing your high school buddies at a reunion or worse, your heart stops while you are working out at the gym. Yikes.

. . . .

I am asking you to explore your most present fears and pain. Like the motivation exercise of finding your 'place of pleasure,' just the thought of your most powerful negatives will have an emotional charge for you. They may be right on the surface or you might have to dig a little further for them. Some might be obvious – for example, you have identified one or more food intolerances and you know that the outcome of eating those foods is pain (either immediately or within a few hours afterwards). There is value in remembering the pain, as it is easier to say no to the offending culprits. For me, in my wheat and dairy intolerant phase a few years back, I would only have to remind myself of the bloating and spasms to find the motivation to not eat my favourite foods of bread and cheese.

Now go ahead, write down the pain of being overweight, of not being healthy. It can be physical, emotional, mental, or spiritual.

What will be the outcome in one year from now if nothing changes – if in fact, you continue to gain weight rather than lose it?

Now imagine it. Feel it. See it. Let it move you to take action. Capture your imagination of being in the 'place of pain' so that you can make use of it, as needed. There may be moments that your pain works more effectively than your pleasure. You may want to give it a personal name as you did the other. Georgia, the mother who was motivated by being a role model for her daughter called her painful place, 'Fat Mother.'

Whatever motivates, or inspires you – it needs to be yours. It needs to be real and true for you because losing weight and getting healthy will not happen if you do it for any other reason than for yourself. Indirectly, you know it will affect the ones you love in a positive way and clearly that is a good thing that may be an added source of inspiration. However, it won't be enough if you don't connect with the reasons that matter to you. No hounding by your doctor, sway by the media, taunting by strangers, suggestions by friends is going to get you to do what you need to do to be healthy and light if you don't feel, right down to your bones, an internal motivation to do so.

Week #2

• • • • • • • • • • • • • • • •

Eat Breakfast and Continue Eating

• • •

Be Accountable to Someone Other than Yourself

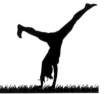

Eat Breakfast and Continue Eating

What you need to do

Eat breakfast.

Then keep eating every three hours. (Okay, it might be every two to four hours, but let's make it simple and call it 'three' for now. Later you can refine that to your personal metabolism.)

Include protein and fibre at each meal.

Why you need to do it

James O. Hill, PhD, is co-founder of the National Weight Control Registry, which monitors the habits of people who have lost a minimum of thirty pounds and have kept it off from one to sixty-six years. What he and his colleagues have discovered is that the route to weight loss varies widely, yet sustaining a good weight has some commonalities. One of those is eating breakfast. Seventy-eight percent of successful losers eat breakfast every day and ninety percent eat it five days per week. This makes sense from a physiological standpoint: Eating breakfast breaks the nighttime fast and tells your body that it is time to get the metabolism revved up for the day. Not eating breakfast keeps you in 'famine mode.' In this state, your brain and body assume that you have no access to energy from food. Your body responds by lowering its energy expenditure. In the process, calorie burning slows down. The other consequence of famine mode is that it leads to intense cravings later in the day, particularly for carbs, sugar and fatty foods.

Eating every three hours starting with a breakfast which includes protein and fiber, helps to stabilize those hormones that play a role in freeing sugar from the fat cells to be burned for fuel. Recall the discussion in last week's chapter. Protein catalyzes the release of the hormone glucagon, which is needed for the fat cells to shrink as well as blood sugar stability between meals.

Fibre also contributes to blood sugar stabilization and a more complete sense of fullness and satiation. A research review at Jean Mayer USDA Human Nutrition Research Center on Aging at Tufts University highlighted that when overweight individuals added 14 grams of fibre daily to their otherwise unrestricted diet, they consumed ten percent fewer calories. This led to an average of 4.2 pounds of weight loss in just under four months

The brain and body need a constant and steady supply of fuel and nutrients. If you don't provide them consistently throughout the day you set yourself up for unstable moods, low energy, and difficulty in achieving and maintaining your weight loss. The mid-afternoon lull in energy is evidence of this. Along with fatigue, you may be struck with an inability to concentrate, an intense desire for something sweet and the need for a cup of coffee to keep you going. Later, hours after your hit of stimulants, you then encounter potent nighttime cravings. Given the prevailing tendency to have a long stretch of five to eight hours between lunch and dinner, the first line of defense against mid-afternoon and evening cravings is to eat a snack around three or four o'clock. Otherwise you're not feeding enough nutrients to your brain nor maximizing your body's natural metabolic capacity.

Finally, if you think that you can make up for your lack of meals throughout the day by consuming copious amounts of calories in the evening, think again. Although there is a diet trend promoting the idea of daytime fasting followed by consumption of the bulk of calories consumed in a four-hour window at night, there is little solid research to support this. Most people are neither prepared physically nor psychologically for daytime fasting, nor would it serve them in a sustainable way.

How you can do it

The idea that we can be healthy and light by eating a boxed cereal every morning is a testament to the brilliance of marketing and how that marketing weaves its way into the human psyche. If you look at the ingredients of cereals, you'll notice that they are low in protein plus high in carbs and sugar. This isn't conducive to optimal health, nor a sustainable loss of fat.

Instead, go back to your list of proteins and decide which ones you would be willing to eat in the morning. It doesn't have to be limited to the standards of egg, dairy and whole grains but if that is what you prefer and are comfortable with, there are certainly some good options.

In addition to protein, you'll also need to include fibre, which is abundant in vegetables, fruit, beans, whole grains, seeds and nuts. However keep in mind that protein is acidic and we need an accompaniment of alkaline foods to keep our tissues in a healthy state. The only fibrous foods that are alkalizing are vegetables and fruit. Vegetables are a better companion for most proteins, and are also lower in sugar content, so they should be your fibre of choice for a minimum of two meals, if not more. (More on vegetables, fruit, acid and alkaline in week #5, *Fall in Love with Vegetables*). I also recommend the addition of one to two tablespoons of ground flax or chia seed to breakfast or another meal. Both seeds are high in the much needed Omega 3 fats (more on this in week #7, *Eat Good Fats, Get Rid of the Bad*) and soluble fibre. Aim for a total of around 35 grams of fibre per day across all meals and snacks. (Most of the North American population is getting only 11 - 15 grams per day.)

You will find some breakfast options below. My suggestion is to find three breakfasts that you like and alternate them during your workweek. The weekend may be an opportunity to prepare a dish that takes more time and might be a bit more indulgent.

- **Protein Shakes** – An excellent option for those of us who don't want to eat heavily in the morning and want something quick and nutritious. Check out the recipes on my site www.foodcoach.ca for a variety of shake recipes that are delicious. Once you have practiced them a few times, they are quick and easy to make. You can also include all kinds of nutritious but weird tasting powders, like 'supergreens' and medicinal mushroom combos that would otherwise be challenging to consume.

* **Hot cereal–** Steel cut oats, rolled oats, or a mixture of grains that includes amaranth and/or quinoa. Add nuts or seeds, your favorite milk, some cinnamon or nutmeg, and stevia, or a small amount of another quality sweetener. Or eat it savory with a little flax oil, hemp oil, or coconut oil and tamari (naturally aged Japanese soy sauce) or herbal sea salt. Optionally, you can steam some leafy greens into it in the last few minutes. Up the protein by combining it with Greek yogurt, boiled eggs or protein powder.

* **Eggs –** An omelet or scrambled (using coconut or avocado oil to fry on medium heat), poached, or boiled – mix with any of feta or ricotta or another cheese, vegetables, lots of herbs (basil, cilantro, dill and parsley are all nice). Serve with leafy green or raw vegetables and whole grain toast or beans. If you are in a hurry, boiling eggs while you're doing other things makes it fast and easy. Or making hard-boiled eggs the night before, makes for a quick grab at breakfast or as a snack later in the day.

* **Yogurt or Cottage or Ricotta cheese –** A mixture of apples or berries and other fruit with yogurt (plain, preferably Greek for the higher protein, and natural – only milk and bacterial culture) or kefir along with raw nuts and seeds. Optionally, cottage or ricotta cheese with fruit or vegetables and roasted sesame seeds or herbs on top.

* **Protein Pancake –** delicious and filling with lots of protein. I make up a batch of the dry ingredients and divide it to last for four breakfasts. Then preparation is five minutes and another fifteen to cook while you do other things. The recipe can be found on my website at www.foodcoach.ca.

* **Seed and Fruit Cereal –** This was inspired by a couple of prepared cereals that can be found in health food stores, but you can make it easily for a fraction of the cost. It's a mixture of chia and hemp seeds, raw buckwheat groats, cinnamon, natural sea salt, dried blueberries, and coconut flakes. I have posted a recipe on my site. I call it 'Chia Wonder Cereal.' You can adapt it, as you like. I soak it in almond milk for a few minutes, add pomegranate seeds or other fruit, and Greek yogurt. Filled with fibre, rich in Omega 3

fats. Make sure you drink lots of water throughout the day (see next week) to maximize the benefit of the fibre.

Once breakfast is taken care of, the most common challenge is what to eat for the mid afternoon snack. To that end, here is another list, this one focused on some healthy and well-balanced options for that meal between breakfast and lunch and/or lunch and dinner. The same principles apply. Your snack is a mini meal that needs to include protein and fibre.

- Cottage cheese, ricotta cheese or Greek yogurt with fruit and nuts/seeds
- Mexican lettuce roll-up – refried beans, avocado, salsa, cheese, hot spice, sprouts (or any configuration of these) rolled in lettuce
- Vegetables with hummus or another bean dip
- A colorful selection of raw vegies – carrots, celery, cucumber, red pepper, broccoli, jicama, cherry tomatoes with a slice of cheese, ricotta or cottage cheese
- Sardines (or another fish) mixed with olive oil, lemon and sea salt and pepper, stuffed into celery sticks
- Almond or sesame butter on rice crackers or on veggies such as carrots or celery
- A protein powder shake or a meal replacement such as *Natural Factors Slimstyles* (www.naturalfactors.com) or *Vega One* (www. myvega.com)
- Green smoothie with a hit of protein powder in it. You will find the recipe on my site.
- Smoked salmon and cream cheese on cucumbers
- Prosciutto (or other high quality meat slices) wrapped around cheese and veggies
- Hard-boiled eggs with vegetables
- Protein bars – some are better than others. Look for ones that are free of health-depleting ingredients, such as hydrogenated or partially hydrogenated fats and chemical sweeteners. They also need to have a relatively high amount of protein (Ideally, a minimum of 15 grams) to counter the always-high carbohydrate component. A higher fibre, lower sugar content is a bonus.

Be Accountable to Someone Other Than Yourself

What you need to do

If you have, many times over, made promises to yourself to change your eating or to exercise more, and have not been able to stick with it, relax. You are not alone. Breaking long-standing patterns of inactivity and comfort eating takes focus and commitment. Doing it alone can be confusing and overwhelming.

Imagine how different it would be if you had at least one person supporting you through the whole process. Someone who could help you determine the next step that you have to take, and who you would check in with on a weekly basis. No bull, just the truth. No judgment, only unconditional support.

Whether it is a friend, family member, work colleague, coach or a live or online group, it is important to find others who will support you and to whom you can offer the same. These are your buddies or buddy group. This week is focused on figuring out who, what, when and how you can get extra encouragement to help you make it through the challenges of changing your patterns.

Why you need to do it

It is human nature (and the nature of our human brain) to take the easy and most familiar road. Accountability to another increases your chance of choosing the more challenging and less familiar route until it becomes habit, improving the likelihood that you'll succeed. We are more likely to follow through if we know someone else is expecting something of us.

> *Barb, my client who had gone back to work after raising her kids, had a habit of committing to going to the gym, but not following through. The appeal of getting home to hang out with her husband, have dinner and watch TV would over-take her when she was low in energy at the end of the day. She discovered that a co-worker was struggling with similar issues, so they became gym buddies. They negotiated on the fitness classes that they would go to and made plans to meet each other there. Neither wanted to let the other one down. In six months Barb ended up missing only three classes. By then, she was hooked, so when her buddy had some personal issues that made it difficult to continue going at that time of the day, Barb kept going on her own.*

Barb's not alone in her need for a buddy. The human brain is wired to do what's easiest, especially when we're tired, under stress, or learning new things. Well-worn pathways form in our nervous system when we have practiced something over and over again. This creates the ease of auto-mation. On the other hand, new habits have yet to entrench their pattern through the neural network. If going for a workout or eating a protein salad for lunch is not already an oft-repeated practice, and therefore automated, it is just too easy to say 'no' to the healthier choice. Bring in one or more other people however, make a commitment to them and you have now engaged your 'social brain' in your decision-making. Research shows that when we collaborate towards a goal, we are more likely to succeed. When your social brain is engaged you have a better chance of following through on your plans.

Think of a past New Year's resolution where your determination seemed fierce in the moment but was short-lived. According to an online experiment led by psychologist Richard Wiseman at The University of Hertfordshire, seventy-eight percent of people will fall off their resolutions before the year is up. What we're after is sustainability; so any engaging tool you can use to your advantage will increase your likelihood of success. Accountability is one of them.

How you can do it

The nature of a buddy relationship is that it will have its own nature. Creating an influential buddy system requires you to be thoughtful about your needs.

Be clear about your motivation.

This was covered in week one, but it's important to reflect on your internal and external motivations so that you have clarity about why you would look for a buddy in the first place.

Articulate your challenges.

Say them out loud and write them down so you are clear about what you need help with. Then think about who or what kind of a buddy system will work best for you based on those challenges. Whichever you choose, it needs to be supportive of your goals and motivation, and non-judgmental about your challenges.

Determine the best buddy system for you

Here are some of the pools of buddy opportunities:

- Friend, family or co-worker
- Health and weight loss coach

- Personal trainer
- Live groups and classes
- Online groups
- Tracking system

As in all relationships, the buddy relationship is one of give and take. It is helpful to know not only what you need but also what you can give in return. Maybe you have lots of money but not much time, in which case, hiring a professional coach or trainer might make the most sense. On the other hand, you may be more flexible with your time, so a group class is doable. Energy may be more of what you have to give so an online support group or a friend would be better suited to your buddy system. Maybe you're not quite ready to engage another person in your process, so a tracking system is where you would like to start.

Communicate with your buddy

You've figured out what your motivation, challenges and needs are. Now communicate them. Talk about how you're going to support each other. Here are some ideas (some may apply only to a one-on-one relationship and some work better in a group setting):

- Establish personal weekly goals and commit verbally to each other
- Work out together
- Share recipes and resources
- Share ideas and tips about things that work for you
- Brainstorm ways that you can overcome an obstacle
- Pass on information when one person misses a session
- Call on each other for support when you are facing a challenge
- Push each other when you are lacking motivation
- Have a friendly competition
- Pass on information to the group via your buddy when you aren't able to attend a session

Talk ahead of time about how you see your buddy being helpful to you when you are stuck. Stay in conversation with your buddy about what's happening. It's so much easier when you can get out of your own head to realize that you are not alone in your challenges.

Consider Food Tracking

Research has shown that tracking what you're eating can increase your success rate.

A 2008 study coordinated by the Kaiser Permanente Center for Health Research in Portland involving 1,685 people over a six-month period, found that those who consistently tracked their food, lost double the amount of weight than those in the study who didn't. This is because people tend to underestimate the amount that they're eating. Tracking keeps you honest with yourself and offers another tool to increase your accountability with others. It can also be insightful to see quantities by way of calories, protein, carbs, fat, sugar and fibre. The numbers can make over-consumption, or for that matter, under-consumption more obvious. I have witnessed the shock value that it has for people. It can lead to an 'ah-ha' moment where they can now see what they couldn't see before. Tracking gives you insight not only to the quantity of food but helps add to your understanding of the positive and negative effect that particular food might have on your weight loss efforts.

However there are some drawbacks and it would be valuable to keep them in mind. Tracking programs demonstrate a limited perspective on food. They are designed to focus on the numbers: calories and the macronutrients (protein, fat and carbs). They don't reflect the nutritional quality of what you're eating nor how well it will be utilized in your body.

For those who have a history of being obsessed with food and the numbers associated with it, I would suggest that you move away from tracking and focus your attention in other areas such as paying attention to your body signals. Learning to relax and enjoy food will be a far more powerful balance in your movement towards sustainability.

Use tracking, if you need to, in the initial stages of change to get a sense of the caloric cost and nutrient profile of the foods that you're eating, and to be realistic with your intake. Learn from it and then let it go. You can always return to it again if it helps you to keep yourself in check.

A few notes of caution

Buddies are there to keep each other moving forward. Be cautious of using the buddy system as a way to waste time that could be better used to reach your goals, like getting exercise or prepping meals.

Angelie was a woman in one of my group classes who was now going to the gym with her sister four days per week. Despite the increase in frequency of exercise, her progress seemed particularly slow. She commented that she wasn't seeing any results in terms of weight loss or strength gains. It turns out that she and her sister would get on the treadmill beside each other and maintain a slow enough speed (essentially walking) so they could talk throughout their hour. After a discussion with the group, Angelie decided to talk with her sister about doing their 'walk and talk' two days per week – they didn't want to give them up entirely because they really enjoyed talking to each other and this was the best time to do it. She would suggest that on the other days, they could meet at the beginning of their workout to determine what challenges each was going to take on and then they would catch up at the end to discuss their workouts. Her sister agreed. From that point on, Angelie came to the group sessions with far more energy and excitement because she had a balanced plan to help her reach her goals.

If you are choosing a professional coach or personal trainer, look for someone that you feel comfortable with, and who seems to be able to give you what you need. Also make sure that they walk their talk. Choose a person who has already done what you are trying to do and seems to be able to communicate their approach in a way that you can relate to. You also need to have a sense that they are totally in it for your success. If you don't feel that wholeheartedly from a pro, choose someone else.

Week #3

. . . .

Commit to Upping Your Water Intake

. . .

Stop Beating Yourself Up

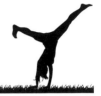

Commit to Upping Your Water Intake

What you need to do

Up your water intake. Start with increasing the amount you're drinking by one glass per day and work up from there. Eventually, you'll need to aim for your personal ideal based on the numbers to follow.

People often mention that water is a problem for them. They don't think about it or they don't like it. I get it. It hardly ranks high on the flavor scale and if you don't have it readily available, it isn't something that you are likely to think much about in a busy day.

For some of you however, this will be the 'low hanging fruit', the easiest thing that you can grab onto to create change. For others, it is a bigger challenge. Either way, take it one step at a time. If you struggle with drinking water use some of the tips that are suggested in the 'how to do it' section to make water consumption easier and eventually, habitual.

Why you need to do it

"The muscles that move your body are approximately seventy-five percent water; the blood that transports nutrients is eighty-two percent water; the lungs that provide your oxygen are ninety percent water; the brain that is the control center of your body is seventy percent water; even your bones are twenty-two percent water." * Water regulates all functions of the body. So doesn't it make sense that it would have its effects on how our body manages its weight loss and weight gain? Absolutely.

Drinking enough water ranks high in the top five list of the most important shifts you can make in your nutrition to be healthy and light. The involvement of water in every aspect of the body's functioning, including weight loss, cannot be underestimated.

The brain needs a constant supply of fuel to meet its energy needs. It gets that from glucose (the simplest form of sugar) and from water in the form of 'hydroelectric power' (much like a hydro station built on a dam that generates power for the surrounding area). In an effort to get fuelled, the brain sends out hormonal messengers that signal hunger. In moments nearing energy deficiency, those signals will show up as cravings for sugar, which provides a quick source of fuel. If you drink water instead, you can curtail the desire to eat sugar as the brain is now, at least for the moment, having its energy needs satisfied.

You may wonder why you are rarely thirsty if you need so much water. Our sensations for hunger and thirst are intricately tied together in a small but mighty part of the brain called the hypothalamus. As a result, a need for water can be misinterpreted as a signal for food. In someone who doesn't routinely drink water, chances are good that they have learned to ignore the subtle signals of thirst. For those people, by the time they get to a thirsty state, they are already dehydrated. In addition, the physiology of thirst is dependent on water itself. Without it, you have turned off the efficiency of the thirst pathway that would signal you to drink. A consistent supply of water ensures that the thirst signals are working proficiently. You will then also be aware of the subtle sensations that suggest a need to drink.

Drinking enough water can have the powerful effect of reducing your appetite, increasing your digestive power, stabilizing your moods, helping you to deal with stress better, and increasing your energy. All of these results are contributing factors for weight loss.

It may seem like a lot of power to give to the humble fluid, but consider the research done by Dr. Batmanghelidj who has studied the effects of the lack of water on our body and its disease states for over 30 years. Weight loss, diabetes, arthritis, chronic pain, stress, high blood pressure, high cholesterol, heart disease, asthma and allergies, insomnia and even AIDS are some of the dysfunctions that he claims are, at least in part, dehydration issues. He backs each up with an understanding of the metabolic pathways affected by lack of water, supportive research, as well as reflections from patients that he has helped by having them rehydrate.

It's a 'no-brainer'. Chances are good that you need to drink more water.

How you can do it

How much should you drink?

The general rule is to drink (in ounces) half your weight (in pounds). So if you weigh 200 pounds, drink 100 ounces of water each day. If you think in metric, it's 14 ml. per pound of body weight.

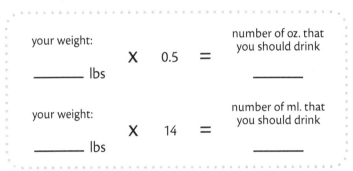

your weight: _____ lbs $\times$ 0.5 = _____ number of oz. that you should drink

your weight: _____ lbs $\times$ 14 = _____ number of ml. that you should drink

Another sure way to know if you are getting enough water is to observe your urine. It should be clear or very light yellow in color. A deeper color indicates dehydration.

First morning pee is usually dark in color because of the lack of water available throughout the night. So guess what you should do first thing in the morning before you consume anything else, including coffee? You got it – drink a minimum 10 – 12 ounce (300 – 350 ml) glass of water.

How can you help yourself to drink more water?

The aim is to make it easy and automatic for you to drink consistently throughout the day.

Here are some ideas that may help:

- Measure out your water intake for the day and fill a pitcher so you can keep track of your progress.

- Keep the pitcher of water and a glass on your desk or wherever you spend most of your day. Seeing it will be a reminder to drink.

- Carry a stainless steel water bottle with you wherever you go and as often as you can. Every time you look at it, take a drink.

- Add lemon, cucumber, orange, watermelon, mint, chlorophyll (I use one with natural mint flavoring), or a small amount of a favorite herbal tea to your water to increase its taste satisfaction.

- Drink a glass of water before each meal and after each meal as a consistent structure and to reduce appetite.

- As mentioned, you need to start every day with at least one tall glass of water. You may want to add the juice of half a lemon. This not only ensures that you start the day off on a good note of hydration but the phytochemical d-limonene in lemon supports liver detoxification.

What type of water is best?

If you are not drinking enough, any water will do. Don't get too hung up on the purification of water if all you can get is tap water. Having said that, if you have access to a reliable source of spring or natural mineral water, or to water purified by reverse osmosis or distillation, go for it. This is more likely to offer cleaner water that is free of volatile organic chemicals, radioactive substances, and additives such as chlorine, fluoride and flocculents. Make sure you are getting enough natural sea salt and minerals from plant based foods in your diet, to compensate for the lack of minerals in the reverse osmosis and distilled water and for the flushing out of minerals from your body.

Watch out for bottled water. You may prefer the taste and the convenience, but the environmental cost of trashed bottles is exorbitant. Also you are often paying for water that is just filtered tap water. There are far fewer government regulations on the bottled water industry than there are on our municipal tap sources. Municipal water is tested daily. Bottled water companies are sometimes not tested for years running.

Also be extra cautious of flavored waters. Most have either sugar or chemical sweeteners, such as Splenda (sucralose), acesulfame K or aspartame – all of which will defeat the purpose of drinking water in the first place. In fact the chemical sweeteners are linked to increases in appetite and obesity.

Do other fluids and foods count towards your water intake?

That depends.

Herbal teas could be included in your total water count. Also if you are eating your six full servings of vegetables every day, or drinking broth-based soups, you probably won't need as much water. Truth is, most foods and beverages contain some water and ultimately could be counted within your total water intake (TWI) for the day. However, the TWI is far more than I am suggesting here. Even the conservative Institute of Medicine recommends a minimum of 3.7 L and 2.7 L for healthy men and women, respectively. Those amounts would increase with more activity, hotter temperatures, more sweating and higher fat levels. Fat contains less water than lean muscle mass, so you have to make up for the lower total body water percentage by upping your intake. To summarize, yes other fluids and foods count, but they do so in the context of even higher needs than I have recommended. So, let's go back to drinking half your weight in **water** alone to ensure adequate hydration.

What about coffee and other caffeinated beverages? A 2004 review of the scientific literature by the Institute of Medicine, states that in healthy individuals, the intake of caffeinated beverages does have a positive effect on hydration. However, I see a lot of people in my practice who have overtaxed adrenals, the glands that help us adapt to stress. Stimulation from caffeine can potentially deplete the adrenals more than they already are. This will not serve your health or weight loss efforts. Therefore, although it is possible that coffee may not be dehydrating and might even contribute to your hydration, don't count it as part of your water supply.

Can you get too much water?

Anything taken beyond moderation, into extremes, can have a detrimental effect. That would include obsessive water intake. Too much water can dilute the sodium concentration of the blood and cause swelling in tissues that expand to offer cellular storage space for water. However, let's be clear. We're talking about huge quantities of water, beyond what many people would drink in a week, never mind a day. Consider that one healthy kidney can excrete between 700 ml and 1000 ml of water in just one hour. Which means that two kidneys could do double that. At those rates, you could drink a lot of water in a day without much concern for dilution or swelling. If you keep your intake to what is suggested here, then you'll be doing well.

If, on the other hand, you happen to be a marathon runner or other long endurance athlete, then you would have to monitor your fluid intake closely. During the physical stress of intense exercise, the kidneys cannot excrete excess water.

Otherwise, it is important to make sure that you are balancing your water intake with enough electrolytes – potassium, calcium, magnesium, sodium and chloride. If you eat enough natural plant based foods, and include a moderate amount of Himalyan, Celtic (or other sun-dried) sea salt to your diet (½ teaspoon for 70 ounces or 2 litres of water in a day,) all should be well.

For most of us, the biggest issue is that we have to pee more.

Let the need to go to the bathroom be an excuse to get up from your desk (or otherwise) and walk more.

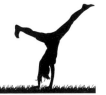

Stop Beating Yourself Up

What you need to do

Stop beating yourself up. Instead, practice seeing yourself in a positive light. Look for what functions well, what is good, and what is beautiful. If you are open and willing, the positive energy will provide you with the abundant resources you need to take care of yourself and to fuel your transformation.

This may be a tough one because we, as a population, suffer a common affliction. It's the 'not good enough' syndrome. Whether we've identified it or not, few of us are immune to its affects. For women, we face a barrage of 'not enoughs': not beautiful enough, not smart enough, not lovable enough, not thin enough, not a good enough mother, not sexy enough, not caring enough, not popular enough, on and on and on it goes. Men face their own versions of 'not good enough'. Not a good enough man, provider, lover, partner, not good enough at his work, not competent enough. There are many versions of the 'not enough' syndrome. It is inherent in our human nature to focus on what is negative rather than positive.

This week is about taking a deep breath, and shifting your focus towards love. It's about discovering ways to talk to yourself that are kind, caring and resultantly energizing. First you'll need to notice your self-talk, and then you'll practice switching it to a perspective about what is good about you and what you are grateful for.

Why you need to do it

Dopamine, the feel good hormone that gives us motivation and drive, floods our body when we are in a positive state. Positive thinking naturally makes us happier and turns on the learning centers in the brain so that we are able to take on new challenges and be successful at them.

The abundance of dopamine and corresponding energy gives us more internal resources to do what we need to do to take care of ourselves.

It seems simple enough to focus on the positive, but experience tells us that it's easier said than done.

A woman that I'll call Serita came in for one of her weekly sessions. As soon as the door closed, she piped out, "I'm such a bad eater". Her tone of voice and the slouch in the chair displayed her discouragement. When we reviewed her week, I could see that she had eaten extremely well on six days. However, on one day, she had spent time with her mother, who has a judgment about Serita's weight and a tendency to suggest whatever extreme diet she has most recently come across. By the time Serita left the company of her mother she felt depleted. Her thoughts were focused on how fat she was and that she may never be able to lose weight. It was then that she reached for her comfort foods of choice: pizza and fries. As we reviewed the week, Serita was able to see how she had focused on the one bad day rather than all the other days that she had done so well.

Psychological studies demonstrate that as humans we have a propensity to focus on the negative rather than the positive – so much so that researchers have given it a label. It's called *positive-negative asymmetry*. This asymmetry may be explained in part by our survival mechanisms and the need to be attentive to potential threat. However for the sake of transforming our body, we need to learn to focus on the good.

The problem with looking for the negative is that it drains your energy. You can test this out by saying to yourself "I am fat" or "I have no willpower" or any other commonly repeated negative thought that you claim as true. Notice what it feels like in your body when you say it. Does it give you lots of energy, so much so that your next move is to make a salad for yourself or go for a run?

> *I was working with a client who said, "I am fat" as though it were an absolute. She is a marathon runner, a cyclist and a lover of all forms of exercise, so you can probably understand when I say that she is far from fat. She looks strong and athletic to me but in her mind she thinks that she's fat. As soon as she said it, I asked her to close her eyes and notice what is happening in her body. "It zaps my energy and makes me want to eat."*

Focusing on the positive on the other hand, can bring an immediate flush of energy and insight. In Serita's case, when she made the shift to focus on the fact that she had eaten well six out of seven days, her energy perked up and she sat up straighter. That was when she got insight into how her mother triggers her and what she can do about it next time so that she doesn't get so easily derailed. The positive thinking flooded her with the internal resources she needed to move forward rather than staying stuck.

There is another association that comes naturally when you stop beating yourself up. You develop a capacity to forgive yourself. If you want to be healthy and light, you have to let go of the weight of self-judgment and replace it with self-compassion and forgiveness. How much better would you feel if you were able to use your capacity for kindness towards others, for yourself as well?

Now, I know what some of you are thinking: "If I forgive myself, I'll be giving in to my weakness and I'll lose my motivation to try harder." This is boot camp mentality and it works in some situations some of the time, but not in all situations all of the time, nor over the long term. Research shows that forgiveness improves our overall sense of wellbeing, reduces chronic pain, improves cardiovascular risk outcomes, and leads to a reduced likelihood of substance abuse (including food).

How you can do it

To 'stop beating yourself up' you need a shift in perspective, attention, and brain chemistry. It might sound like a lot of work to do all that, but it comes down to some simple steps. Those steps are based on creating 'a practice'. This is a practice rooted in self-compassion, self-love, and self-forgiveness.

Remember one of the underlying principles of *Jump Off the Diet Treadmill* – **whatever you practice you will get better at**. Practice beating yourself up, you'll get better at beating yourself up. Practice seeing yourself in a positive way, you'll get better at it. Practice seeing yourself from a place of love and you will feel more love. Practice compassion and forgiveness and you will be better at compassion and forgiveness.

The reason that practice is so important is that it strengthens the neural pathways in your brain and your entire nervous system. Strong neural pathways are a result of habits, those things that you do over and over again without even thinking about it. Strong neural pathways also mean that something will be easy for you to repeat. Right now, if you tend towards beating yourself up, then you have strong pathways in your body that support that and make it easy. To change an old habit that no longer serves you to reach your goals, you need to replace it with a good habit that does help you reach your goals. That is why we have to practice. And practice. And practice some more.

In week #1, you discovered what motivates you externally and internally and you found your 'place of pleasure'. Now is the time to apply it for the sake of this practice of self-love.

For every moment that you can catch yourself beating yourself up for one thing or another that you did or didn't do, call yourself on it. State it clearly

– "I am beating myself up" so there is no doubt in your mind that you might be doing otherwise. Then, you have some options – one is to replace your negativity with the vision that you have of yourself in your 'place of pleasure.' Alternatively, you can think of something else that is positive and true about you. Consider what you do well, what fine character traits you have, what is beautiful about you. You can always find something positive if you look for it. It is just a shift in focus and a choice to bring your attention to it.

You can make good use of gratitude as well. What are you grateful for? In any given moment, there is an abundance of potential grace. Think of how well your body functions. (See week #9 – *Create a Healthy Relationship with Your Body* for more on this). Show yourself some love. Verbally acknowledge what is beautiful about you.

Being positive is as simple as a shift of what you pay attention to. The act itself is not difficult but it does take practice. Initially, like all things that we are unpracticed at, it will be unfamiliar territory and it may seem awkward. It might even seem a wee bit untrue. Keep working on it. Find what is true and loving. It will seem easier with time and repetition.

Greg was about thirty pounds above what he considered his ideal weight when he came to work with me. He had been training in the gym three days per week for about three months. He was getting stronger but still couldn't seem to shed much fat. Every time he looked in the mirror, he hated what he saw. With me consistently touting the necessity to stop beating himself up, he finally took note to 'be kind to self.' On a return session I noticed that he seemed lighter. Something had shifted. Sometime in the previous week, when he was looking in the mirror, instead of narrowing his focus towards the fattest areas of his body, as he tended to do, he flexed his biceps, his quads and did a bit of a Mr. Universe routine. Three things happened: he had a good chuckle, which lightened his mood; he realized that he had made significant gains towards his goal; and he felt energized instead of distraught. He had a personal 'ah-ha' moment. He got it – that perception is a choice and it matters.

Finally, a reminder of another principle – **take it one step at a time**. You won't save yourself from a beating every time, but each effort that you make will make it a little easier the next time. Practicing a positive perspective will eventually shift your view of yourself to one filled with compassion, forgiveness and love.

In the meantime, take the compassion test below to see how much work you need to do in the 'stop beating yourself up' category. Once you get your scores you can see some other ideas on how you can practice self-compassion. Some suggestions will resonate with you and some won't. You don't need to do them all but choose something to practice. All of this is about relinquishing the energy-draining negativity and replacing it with energy-conserving positivity. Then you'll have the vigor that you need to make the physical changes that will ultimately make the biggest difference for your health and your life.

The following questionnaire and insights into developing compassion, are taken from www.self-compassion.org. This is the site of Dr. Kristin Neff, a human development researcher who studies self-compassion. (Reprinted with permission by the author.)

Scoring Your Level of Self-Compassion

Please read each statement carefully before answering. To the left of each item, indicate how often you behave in the stated manner, using the following scale:

Almost Never				Almost Always
1	2	3	4	5

_____ I try to be loving towards myself when I'm feeling emotional pain.

_____ When I'm going through a very hard time, I give myself the caring and tenderness I need.

_____ I'm kind to myself when I'm experiencing suffering.

_____ I'm tolerant of my own flaws and inadequacies.

_____ I try to be understanding and patient towards those aspects of my personality I don't like.

_____ **TOTAL – *Self-Kindness*** (0 – 12 is low, 13 – 17 is moderate, 18 – 25 is high in self-kindness)

_____ I'm disapproving and judgmental about my own flaws and inadequacies.

_____ When times are really difficult, I tend to be tough on myself.

_____ I'm intolerant and impatient towards those aspects of my personality I don't like.

_____ When I see aspects of myself that I don't like, I get down on myself.

_____ I can be a bit cold-hearted towards myself when I'm experiencing suffering.

_____ **TOTAL – *Self-Judgment*** (0 – 12 is low, 13 – 17 is moderate, 18 – 25 is high in self-judgment)

_____ When things are going badly for me, I see the difficulties as part of life that everyone goes through.

_____ When I'm down and out, I remind myself that there are lots of other people in the world feeling like I am.

_____ When I feel inadequate in some way, I try to remind myself that feelings of inadequacy are shared by most people.

_____ I try to see my failings as part of the human condition.

_____ **TOTAL – _Common Humanity_** (0 – 10 is low, 11 – 14 is moderate, 15 – 20 is high in common humanity)

_____ When I think about my inadequacies, it tends to make me feel more separate and cut off from the rest of the world.

_____ When I'm feeling down, I tend to think most other people are probably happier than me.

_____ When I'm struggling, I tend to feel like other people must be having an easier time of it.

_____ When I fail at something that's important to me, I tend to feel alone in my failure.

_____ **TOTAL – _Isolation_** (0 – 10 is low, 11 – 14 is moderate, 15 – 20 is high in isolation)

_____ When something upsets me I try to keep my emotions in balance.

_____ When something painful happens I try to take a balanced view of the situation.

_____ When I fail at something important to me I try to keep things in perspective.

_____ When I'm feeling down I try to approach my feelings with curiosity and openness.

_____ **TOTAL – _Mindfulness_** (0 – 10 is low, 11 – 14 is moderate, 15 – 20 is high in mindfulness)

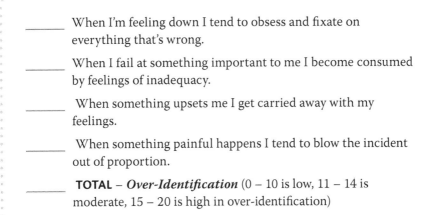

_____ When I'm feeling down I tend to obsess and fixate on everything that's wrong.

_____ When I fail at something important to me I become consumed by feelings of inadequacy.

_____ When something upsets me I get carried away with my feelings.

_____ When something painful happens I tend to blow the incident out of proportion.

_____ **TOTAL** – *Over-Identification* (0 – 10 is low, 11 – 14 is moderate, 15 – 20 is high in over-identification)

Using your scores to identify your biggest gaps in self-compassion, look below for ideas on how to create change in this area.

Self-Kindness – "What would a caring friend say to you in this situation?" "What is a kind and constructive way to think about how I can rectify this mistake or do better next time?" Try putting your hand over your heart or gently stroking your arm when feeling a lot of pain as a gesture of kindness and compassion.

Self-judgment – "Who ever said human beings are supposed to be perfect?" "Would a caring mother say this to her child if she wanted the child to grow and develop?" "How will I learn if it's not okay to make mistakes?"

Common Humanity – Think about all the other people who have made similar mistakes, gone through similar situations, and so on. This is the human condition – all humans are vulnerable, flawed, make mistakes, have things happen that are difficult and painful. "How does this situation give me more insight into and compassion for the human experience?"

Isolation – "I am not the only one going through such difficult times, all people experience things like this at some point in their lives." "Although I take full responsibilities for my mistakes and failings, I also recognize and understand that my actions and behaviors are connected to other people's actions and behaviors – nothing happens in a vacuum."

Mindfulness – Take several deep slow breaths and try to be with your pain exactly as it is. Let yourself feel the pain without suppressing, resisting, or avoiding it. Take a moment to stop and say to yourself, "this is really hard right now." Let yourself be moved and touched by your own pain. Try to see the situation clearly with calm, clarity and a balanced perspective. "I fully accept this moment and these emotions as they are."

Over-identification – Try not to get lost in the drama or storyline of your situation, feel the feelings as they are, without running away with them. Can you feel the emotions in your body (a constriction in your throat, knot in your stomach, etc.) without getting lost in the reason for these feelings? "These difficult emotions do not define me, such feelings will inevitably change and pass away." Don't take your emotions so personally.

Week #4

• • • • • • • • • • • • •

Eat Close to Nature

• • •

Find the Exercise that is Right for You

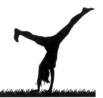

Eat Close to Nature

What you need to do

Eat as close to nature as possible.

Nature, in its finest state, provides the nutrition that we need and helps to protect us from the harmful exposures that we get from our environment.

Eating close to nature is not as easy as it once was, say sixty years ago. Unless we are growing our own food or directly connected to the farmers who are, we are no longer able to consistently buy foods at their finest. We need to become wary travelers of our grocery aisles and marketplaces. We must do our best to take charge of our food where and when we can.

What this means is that you should look for foods that are closest to the form that they were in when they were grown. For example, an apple will be more nutritious than commercial apple juice. Why? The juice is mostly concentrated sugars since the apple fibre and most of its nutrients have been eliminated. It is also likely being stored in a container that may contain aluminum, Bisphenol A or any other number of chemicals used in the manufacture of storage containers.

If the food contains more than one ingredient, choose the ones that have ingredients that you recognize as a food. Yogurt made from just milk and bacterial culture (as it has been done for thousands of years) will have more nutrition than one that includes milk solids, modified milk ingredients (what the heck is that anyway?), cornstarch, or a plethora of other ingredients.

Why you need to do it

Your body and brain are made up of air, water and food. All of those proteins, carbohydrates, essential fats, minerals, vitamins, and enzymes that you have heard about, are transferred from the foods that you eat, via your gastrointestinal tract, to your blood and to the various tissues of your body. The saying that 'you are what you eat' is not far off the mark.* You must get nutrients from your food. If the majority of your food is nutrient-deficient, your body and mind will not function at its best. Nor will you find it easy to be at your ideal weight for any length of time.

The manufacturing of food involves hundreds of different processes, many of which destroy the raw nutrients. Some of the processes not only destroy the good stuff but also add insult to injury by adding in toxic substances as a by-product of the manufacturing itself. The unseen chemicals in the foods that you choose mix with those in your environment to create a dangerous broth that is a likely supporter of fatty tissue. Current research is now focusing on the 'obesogens' that we are exposed to unknowingly. 'Obesogens' is a term coined by biologist Bruce Blumberg from the University of California at Irvine, just one of the researchers bringing attention to this area of 'fat' research. Obesogens are chemicals that disrupt our endocrine system, increasing the probability that we will be obese. They can change how our body responds to calories. These chemicals are common in our food supply, body care products, household chemicals and the rest of our environment. They include BPA (found in the linings of cans, plastic bottles and containers, cash register receipts, etc) and other bisphenols, nicotine, MSG, fructose, and PCB's (abundant in some of the fish we eat), to name just a few. Eating manufactured foods multiplies the effects of obesogens. Not only are you not getting the raw materials that your body needs, but you also amplify the negative effects of the hormone disrupting chemicals. This puts a burden on your detoxification processes and results in a lot of extra storage materials in your fat cells.

Let's dissect a manufactured food to give you an example of the exposure that you could be getting from just that one food. I'll pick on breakfast cereals since I've already bashed them as a source of a healthy breakfast. Now, let's look a little closer. Most of them contain grains that were once whole including the kernel (aka the endosperm), the germ and the bran. The processing of grains used in most cereals, removes the germ and the bran, which extracts the bulk of the fibre, essential omega 3 and 6 fats, the Vitamin E and most Vitamin B's, the minerals and, in many cases, the protein. Many, if not most of the original nutrients are destroyed. That is why you will often discover, when you read labels, that synthetic nutrients have been put back in. This is little comfort, because artificially isolated nutrients do not have the same impact in our body as the naturally occurring nutrients found in foods. In nature, nutrients are never present in isolation. They always have other supportive co-factors that increase the nutrient's availability and effectiveness in the body.

Back to the cereal – what you are left with then, besides synthetic nutrients is a predominance of problematic carbohydrates, i.e. the kind that can potentially make and keep you fat. Adding to the lack of nutrient density is the addition of substances that food manufacturers would rather you didn't know about. Here are just a few of the possible tricks and treats that may be looming in your favorite breakfast cereal:

Hydrogenated or partially hydrogenated fats

You have probably already heard about these. They are a source of trans fats and an increased risk for heart disease.

Food coloring

Red # 40 and Yellow #5 and #6 are the three most widely used food dyes. They have been linked to allergic reactions, behavioral issues in children and contain what could be cancer-causing substances.

Soy lecithin

This is a waste product left over from the processing of soy oil. It is filled with pesticides and solvents. It has been associated with abdominal cramping, diarrhea, menstrual irregularities, allergic reactions and cognitive impairment.

Fructose and high fructose corn syrup (HFCS)

Unlike the naturally occurring fructose contained in fruits, additions of isolated fructose and HFCS are particularly problematic for those looking for weight loss because it can wreck havoc on insulin levels. Twenty-five percent of daily intake of calories from either leads to a higher level of deep belly fat and greater risk for diabetes and heart disease.

BHT and BHA

These are used as food preservatives to decrease the rancidity of fats and increase shelf life. They have been identified as safe in the amount that is in any one food. However, when they accumulate, they may contribute to the damage of red blood cells and stimulate chemical sensitivity. They have also been associated with ADHD in kids and the research is still out on whether tumor-producing molecules within these preservatives might ultimately contribute to the development of cancer.

MSG

This flavoring that is common in Asian cuisine is not limited to eastern cooking. It has found its way into many processed foods in the guise of hydrolyzed or textured vegetable protein (HVP or TVP), protein isolate, calcium caseinate, yeast extract, natural flavors, and seasonings. It has been connected to headaches, respiratory issues and allergic responses in people that are sensitive to it.

I am picking on breakfast cereals here because the marketing for these is so powerful that consumers are lead to believe that they are actually a healthy choice. However we could turn the lens towards almost any food that has been processed, to see that as they get further from their natural state, their benefits are fewer and the dangers greater. Manufactured foods are created using high heat and pressure, chemical solvents, acids and alkalis, heavy metals, and tools and storage containers that are likely to contain residues of toxic or carcinogenic substances.

Edible oils are another example. Oil that is expeller pressed from olives, avocados or coconuts to make an extra virgin oil will be healthier than vegetable or sunflower oil that starts with extraction from the seed using hexane (a solvent made from crude oil processing). After the hexane, it is processed via degumming, refining, bleaching, deodorizing and possibly hydrogenation. All of these processes take out the original vitamins, minerals, fibre, protein, antioxidants and healthy fatty acids. What you have left is a substance that not only has no nutritional value, it is harboring toxic substances that have been linked to heart disease, cancer, diabetes and weight gain. It is, however, cheap. The food manufacturers are counting on you to stay misinformed, and therefore look to pay less for something that you don't realize is contributing to your health issues. (There is a more in-depth discussion of fats in week #6, *Eat Good Fats, Get Rid of the Bad*)

Due to the commercialization of crops, depleted soils, long travel and storage times, harvesting before ripening, and use of pesticides and insecticides, even the simple, unprocessed foods such as vegetables and fruit do not contain the abundant nutrition that they are capable of. Meats, fish, eggs and dairy have their own issues, mostly attributable to the raising of the animals and the preservation of their products.

Just like humans, animals that have higher stress levels, especially when the stress is continuous, will have weaker immunity to infectious organisms and will be more susceptible to spreading those organisms to other animals and humans. The recent salmonella egg recall of five hundred and fifty million factory-farmed eggs in the west and mid-west US, mad cow disease or the swine flu H1N1 are a few well-known cases of infections that traveled beyond the factory.

Consider that an animal or bird that has been raised in a way that is natural to it, where it roams freely, grazes on grass, and experiences normal levels of stress that would be incurred in its natural environment, provides a superior quality of meat, milk and egg than an animal raised under highly stressful and unnatural conditions. Would you rather eat eggs from chickens that have been free roaming outdoors for most of their lives or ones that have been kept in small cages with hundreds of other chickens, their beaks and claws pulled out to prevent them from destroying each other and with an early death looming because of the stressful conditions?

Grass fed, pastured animals have two to four times higher levels of healthy omega 3 fats in their meat and milk, and lower levels of saturated fats than factory farmed animals. The difference can be remarkable; for example,

six ounces of factory-farmed beefsteak can contain eleven grams more total fat than six ounces of the same cut of pasture raised beef. If you were
to change only one thing in your diet – only eating pasture fed animal
products, you would significantly cut down on your unhealthy fat content
which would lend itself to weight loss.

Now that I hopefully have your attention about the issues in the manufacturing of foods, I promise not to leave you hanging in mid-air with an
abundance of negative messages and a concern about what you can eat. The
next section gives you practical info on what you can do to affect positive
change in the quality of your nutrition.

How you can do it

There is always an interesting dichotomy in presenting the nature of food
manufacturing to my clients and groups. On the one hand, it is important
information for people who want to take responsibility for their health.
Those that I share this information with often express gratitude in learning
about it. But it can be overwhelming to consider all of the new choices that
you have to make, where to begin and how to take control. So I will break
this down for you to minimize overwhelm and up the sense of power that
you can get with knowledge.

There is a metaphor about 'low hanging fruit' that is useful at this point.
Pick the fruit that is lowest on the tree and within reach. Go for what is
easiest for you. Choose one processed food that you eat regularly that won't
be hard for you to give up. Decide on what you can replace it with that is
healthy. We will get into more knowledge about best choices as we go further in the program but most people that I've worked with have some sense
of what is healthy and what's not. I suspect you are no different.

*My client Charles, the former athlete and now entrepre-
neur that I introduced you to at the beginning of this book
had been frequenting the food court for lunch, often choosing Asian stir fries with white rice or a sub sandwich. He
knew it would be easy for him to shift his orientation in the*

food court to one of the outlets that had a salad bar where he could load up on vegetables and a protein, like chicken breast or salmon. It is unlikely that the chicken is raised under ideal conditions, that the salmon is wild pacific caught and that the vegetables were organic. But if we imposed those requirements on his lunch it would have drastically limited his choices and overwhelmed him. So happily, he shifted from a poorer quality food choice (fried white rice, sauces with MSG, high heat cooking of the Asian food or high bread content and nitrates in the deli meats of the sub sandwich) to a combination of raw and lightly cooked vegetables and a simple protein source without sauce.

When you are buying packaged foods, read the labels, looking for ingredients that you understand. If you don't know what they are, it is likely that it is a by-product of some kind of processing that has depleted its nutrition. Think about what you could buy that would be a healthier substitute. Turn to week # 11, *Learn to Navigate the Grocery Store* for more direction in choosing better food options.

Prepare as much food from scratch as you have the time and inclination to do. Start with one meal per week that you would otherwise have not done before and add to that slowly and steadily at a pace that you can handle. Make enough for leftovers.

Buy local produce whenever you can. That ensures that it was picked closer to time of ripening than if it had to be shipped from a distance. The longer it is in the ground or on the tree or vine, the more nutritious it will be. It also minimizes the sprays that have to be added to ensure the produce survives the journey. If it is local and organic, even better. Otherwise if you can't get local, buy organic where and when you can.

Look for animal products that are from pasture-raised animals. As mentioned above, their meat, milk, eggs, and cheese will have a higher nutrient content because of the grass that they eat. It is also more humane for the animals. Happy animals make healthier foods. Having said that, it is not easy to find pasture-raised animal foods. It will require some research as to what is available in your area. And free-range does not guarantee that an animal is being raised under truly natural conditions. To find sources of naturally raised animals in your area, check out www.eatwellguide.org .

Not everyone's budget has room for the more expensive organics or pasture-raised animal products, so don't fret it if you can't do it. It's okay. Make the best choices that your time and budget allow for. The key is to take back control of your food to the best of your ability and to do it one step at a time. As your taste buds change (they are very adaptable) and your resolve deepens, you can expand your choices accordingly.

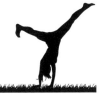

Find the Exercise that is Right For You

What you need to do

Find the exercise that is right for you at this moment in time.

This is not a one-size fits all prescription. What you are ready for, and you will stick with depends on a network of factors. Your work schedule, priorities, starting point, personality, present state of health, lifestyle, mindset, and motivation are all factors in the split seconds that you decide to stick to your exercise commitment or not. Let's go back to one of the principles of this program. *Take it one step at a time.* The point is that you need to get on board with being a 'mover' or if you're already entrenched in an exercise routine, it may be time to take it to the next level.

Why you need to do it

Our bodies were designed to move. Yes, yes even the couch potato body that hasn't moved in years. It's built into our genetic structure.

Flash back to the time when Homo Sapiens and Homo Erectus, our prehistoric cousins, roamed the earth. Scientists' observations tell us that these cousins, that we are 99.9 percent genetically identical to, covered as much as twelve miles per day in search of food and the other necessities of life. Keep in mind that those twelve miles were not on park trails or paved roads. They had to clear forests, traverse savannas, climb mountains, cross deep rivers, fend off saber-tooth tigers and other manner of beast, forage for berries and herbs, trap and kill their food. Time that we spend fixed on our butts in front of a computer or TV they spent in movement. They didn't die of degenerative diseases or get fat.

Much has changed in our world (including a Starbucks or McDonald's on almost every corner) yet little has changed in our genetic structure. Our glorious bodies were created with movement in mind.

We all have heard the facts – exercise is good for your cardiovascular health, the strength of your muscles and bones, the immune system – including reducing the risk of a variety of cancers, as well as diabetes. It helps us sleep, and counters the potential ravages of stress, as well as improving the outcomes for depression and anxiety. In general it makes us feel better, which makes sense since it stimulates the production of the pleasure hormones, dopamine, serotonin and norepinephrine. Exercise increases blood flow to the brain and the rest of the body. Blood is the transport vehicle for oxygen and food nutrients, which means that with exercise your brain and tissues get more of what they need to be nourished and cleansed. Research consistently shows that exercise leads to greater cognitive and problem solving skills as well as an improvement in most kinds of memory. A moving person has more opportunities open to them for change and transformation.

Exercise is good news. But here is the best part: you only need a little to get a lot. In other words, you don't have to wait for the perfect time in your life so that you can make it to the gym four days per week. Your average neighborhood gym counts on a chunk of their revenue coming from people who buy long-term memberships and never show up for more than a few sessions. So don't wait to find just the right time to start an exercise program. That mindset is much the same as the dieter who waits for the periods between holidays and celebrations to go on a diet. Ultimately, this is not the kind of thinking that creates sustainability.

Even twenty minutes of walking or some other kind of daily movement such as gardening or housecleaning creates a positive outcome. It means that as long as you get off your butt and do something, you are moving in the right direction. If you can't handle 20 minutes per day at this point, so be it. Fifteen minutes, three times per week will do too.

I was at a seminar lead by Dr. Len Kravitz, a professor and researcher of exercise science at the University of New Mexico. I was thrilled that he offered some science to back up the notion of movement vs. structured exercise. Dr. Kravitz outlined a research study dividing two groups of self-professed non-exercisers into those who were thin and those who were obese. The thin group moved around in their regular daily activities for two and a half more hours in the day than the obese group. That translates to a calorie burn equivalent to thirty-six pounds per year. The thin people weren't officially exercising, but they were moving.

The point is, get off your butt and do something. Anything more than what you're doing now is a move in the right direction. If you have already established a daily or near daily routine for exercise, good on ya! You may be ready to take it to another level. For those who have yet to confirm themselves as 'movers', keep reading to see how you can make that happen.

How you can do it

For those of you who are already committed to regular exercise, brilliant. Now what is the next step to take it to a higher level? Consider increasing frequency – adding one more day into your routine, shifting to interval training, adding another activity for variance, or bringing play (and thus more joy) into your program. Ask yourself "What do I want from my exercise program?" and "what will take it to the next level?" Remember though, one step at a time. Use the protocol below to help you create a shift.

For those of you who have yet to commit to regular physical activity, let's begin by revising the word from exercise to movement. How can you create more movement in your daily life? Maybe your next step is to walk more stairs instead of taking the elevator, stretching on the floor or riding your stationary bike while you watch TV, dancing to your favorite music while you make dinner, going for neighborhood walks. Get my drift? Not everyone enjoys the routine of the gym workout or long runs. Maybe you have always wanted to learn a particular dance form or how to hula hoop (which is, by the way, an amazing workout). Whatever you decide would work for you my suggestion is to commit to a minimum of three times per week, even if it is for only five minutes each time. If you make your commitment an easy one to achieve, you are more likely to make it happen. The key is to get over the inertia and to avoid the wall of resistance that your mind will create to stop you from taking any action at all. Even though five minutes may not do much physiologically, it will get you off your butt and into movement. Then once you're there, you are more likely to keep going. And as you begin to feel the positive effects that even a little movement can offer to boost your energy, you'll be more likely to increase your commitment over time.

If you are someone who really does not like to exercise, there is nothing physical that you like to do, then I would challenge you to find what you dislike the least and start there. Not liking any exercise has its roots in long-term metabolic imbalances resulting in sluggishness, and often in negative childhood experiences of sports and physical activity. Shift your thoughts from exercise programs to movement, and expand the possibilities to include simple activities (some mentioned above) that will connect you back into your physicality.

What if you have trouble making it a part of your daily life or even doing it three times per week? Well, possibly you haven't been supported to take the right approach. Maybe you chose the wrong exercise for your particular personality, or you took on too much all at once, or your perspective about exercise is skewed.

I want to share a personal story that may offer some value to the importance of finding the right exercise to suit you.

When I was in my mid-twenties, I was twenty pounds overweight. I had grown up playing sports and being active but when I hit puberty, and the emotional roller coaster that went with it, I gained weight and wasn't able to get it off. Despite being a female jock, playing on sports teams at school and riding my bike for transportation throughout my university years, my body held tight to the extra weight. At

26, I decided to pursue a desire that I had had since I was a kid – to become a dancer. Not a performing one – rather someone who was confident dancing in public. I signed up for ballet and jazz classes at the Y but quickly found that I was intimidated by having to follow the steps and leap across the room with everyone watching me. I wasn't comfortable enough in my body to do that. So I quit. But my dance story doesn't end there. I bought a large 4' X 6' mirror and set it up in my spacious room to practice dancing on my own. I discovered my physical calling. I loved dancing freely. I would put on whatever music I was into and dance as I felt like. No steps that I had to follow, no one that I had to impress, I just let go and let my body move. I did whatever felt good no matter how silly it might have looked. It pushed me beyond my self-judgment as well as my flexibility and cardiovascular thresholds. Every night, I would finish my dinner early with the intention to dance and found that I loved the practice – so much so that I continue to do it to this day, 26 years later. I also lost the extra twenty pounds in three months and never gained more than a few pounds back over the years. There is something about the combination of freedom, creativity, connection to the music and letting my body take over my mind that has made this form of 'exercise' work for me. It has also been the most powerful source of emotional release, which makes sense if you consider that emotional memory is stored in tissues throughout the body. Movement stimulates an increase in blood flow to these tissues, which means greater access to the information that is stored. (See week # 7, Take Charge of Your Emotions, for more on this). I still love riding my bike, walking and will get into the gym once per week, but free dance is the foundation that I always return to.

What I have gleaned from my own experience is that everyone will have some form of movement that is more suited to their personality type. Suzanne Brue has written a book on fitness personalities that emphasizes this point. You can take the test to find out what type you are, at her site at www.the8colorsoffitness.com. You'll need to account for your exercise personality when you are considering what routine you can establish for yourself.

Another thing to contemplate is the environment that you find most inspiring to workout. Some people love the gym environment. Others can't stand being in the gym but love being in nature. Still others prefer the quiet calm of a yoga studio or their home space.

Your PEP talk is what will be the core of your Personal Exercise Prescription. It will generate the program that is most likely to help you succeed.

Use past experience to answer the following questions.

* What are some simple ways that you can incorporate more movement into your daily routine? (i.e. taking the stairs, walking part or all the way to work, walking to your colleagues desks rather than emailing them, stretching at your desk).

One of my clients admitted that she sits at her desk and computer for eight hours straight, getting up only to once or twice in the day to go to the bathroom. She wouldn't even leave her desk for lunch. Someone she works with fondly teased her about her attachment to her desk. From our brainstorming, she decided to program a Tweety Bird alarm on her computer every hour. When the bird chirps, it is a reminder to get up and walk around. It worked. She rarely misses her hourly striding – she finds it helps her focus on her work and to problem solve. Her co-worker has been inspired and sometimes joins her on her walks around the office.

- What type of exercise/movement do you enjoy?
- What environment is most inspiring for you to exercise/move in (i.e. anywhere outside, in nature, in a gym, in a yoga studio, in your home)?
- Ideally, whom do you like to exercise with (i.e. alone, one friend, trainer, group)?
- What would you look for in an ideal trainer or teacher?
- Do you like the involvement of other activities (such as talking, watching TV, listening to music) or do you prefer to focus solely on your body and the movement?
- What time of day is best for you to exercise?
- What stops you from exercising/moving on a consistent basis?
- What would help you get over what is stopping you?
- What movement and/or exercise are you willing to commit to for the next week? (Start from where you are at and be realistic with your commitment).
- What do you need to put into place to be accountable to your commitment?

Considering all of the above, create a PEP talk for yourself by filling in the blanks on the next page.

I am committed to doing a minimum of _____ minutes of

_____ ,

at least _____ times this week. The best time for me

to do this is _____ .

I will use _____ to

make it easier to be accountable to this commitment.

If it helps, schedule it into your calendar, get your accountability buddy(s) on board. Do what you need to do to make it happen because once you get yourself moving, you will feel better, you will want to eat better and you be more motivated for the next time. But remember, one step at a time. Only take on what is realistic and what you can stick with. You want to set yourself up for success.

Week #5

Fall in Love with Vegetables

Get in Tune with Your Hunger

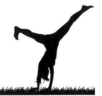

Fall in Love with Vegetables

What you need to do

Include vegetables in your daily 'mealscape'. What this means is that <u>two or more</u> meals each day need to contain a heaping amount of vegetables. Fill at least half of your plate and aim for three different colors at each meal. This adds up to a minimum of six servings of veggies per day. It bears repeating that if this seems like a big task for you, make it simple by aiming for one manageable change at a time. Everything becomes doable when it's broken down into small steps. Keep reading to see how you can make this happen.

Why you need to do it

Vegetables are in the category of 'you don't know what you're missing' until you have them consistently, every day, in abundance. Once you become a vegetable 'seeker', your health goes to an entirely new level. Hitherto unknown feelings of wellness will spring from the roots of your being. Who would have thought foodstuff could inspire such poetics?

Personal experience included, I would sum up how I feel when I get an abundance of vegetables in my day with one word -- light. Light in body and mind. I am more clear and focused, I feel satisfied without being full, my energy is good and I feel balanced. I am not suggesting that I (or you) should eat only vegetables. I need my protein. We all do. But protein without vegetables is like a day without sun. It's less sparkly, even a bit dull. My energy is off, a little out of kilter.

Of all the food groups, only vegetables can boast the combination of minerals, antioxidants, alkalinity, colors, variety of flavors, textures, and the creativity that can be tapped into with such a low caloric cost.

I've harped on the importance of eating so much protein to stimulate the shrinking of your fat cells. There is no better accompaniment to the acidic protein foods than the highly alkalizing vegetable food group. The idea of acid/alkaline balance is to keep our tissues and blood in their narrow pH range. Outside of that range, we either have varying states of disease or we are dead. Arthritis, osteoporosis, tooth decay, immune deficiencies, respiratory issues are just a few examples of acidity gone awry. In general the various food groups tend towards being acidic or alkaline, although some are neutral. Meats, fish, chicken, most grains, beans and legumes, most nuts and seeds, breads, pastas, crackers, cereals, processed foods are acidic. Depending on what chart you consult, most fruits are either neutral or alkaline. The only food group to fit almost exclusively into the alkaline category is sea and land vegetables (with the exceptions of tomatoes and eggplant).

Research on the benefits of the nutrients contained in vegetables, weaves through every body part – from hair to brain to eyes to the heart to the digestive and reproductive organs, to name only a few.

And when it comes to fat loss, research by Dr. Susan Roberts, Professor of Nutrition at Tufts University, indicates that vegetables are the only food group in which you can increase variety and not gain weight. With fruit, the subjects remained neutral, neither gaining nor losing. With all other food groups, there was a correlation between the increase in variety and the amount of weight gained.

Unfortunately most people don't eat enough veggies. If people ate enough, most would be lighter, more emotionally stable, have more energy, and be substantially less at risk for illness and degenerative disease.

From my experience, eating vegetables goes beyond the nutrition research and theories that more than support all the reasons for eating them. It really comes down to creating a renewed terrain in your body and mind.

This is something that you will only get when you try it out. Ultimately you have to have the experience and decide for yourself if vegetables are worth the effort of creating a permanent place for them in your daily mealscape.

How you can do it

Let's be clear -- French fries or a salad made of iceberg lettuce and ranch dressing does not count as a serving of vegetables. But more on that later.

Let's start with how much should you eat.

As mentioned, you will need a minimum of six servings a day. (Check out Week #10, *Take Control of Your Portions* for help with serving sizes.)

Sound like a lot? Well, if you consider that you are eating at least three meals and one to three snacks, there are lots of opportunities to fit them in.

Consider that lunch and dinner and at least one snack should include veggies. And don't veer away from the possibility of eating them at breakfast as well. Nothing goes better with eggs and a slice of whole grain toast (or even better, beans) than a side of raw veggies.

A note about colors: I once created a program called 'Eating in Color' as a reflection of how important it is to increase the colors on your plate at every meal. The general principle is this:

> **Get three different colors of vegetables on your plate at each of two meals, and three different colors of fruit per day. Increase the variety and colors of your spices and herbs.**

The reason for this is to boost the **antioxidant** content of your food intake.

Antioxidants are the first line of defense in your fight against **free radical** damage. Free radicals are unstable molecules that create a domino effect leading to a cascade of damaged tissue. They are the source of, or at least present, in all diseases and injury, as well as the inflammation caused by excess weight.

Free radicals are normally occurring in the body, as are antioxidants. But the onslaught of pollution, stress (this is a big free radical instigator), drugs, and the millions of chemicals that permeate our water, soil, air, and food, increase the damage and our need for more antioxidants.

In comes our HEROS in the fight against free radicals....

Vegetables, fruit, herbs, and spices.

The more colors, the more variety of antioxidants and the deeper the fight against free radicals.

"What if I don't like vegetables?" you ask.

Almost all the people that I have worked with who said that they don't like vegetables, have been able to identify at least five or six vegetables that they do like. If that is the case for you, start with the ones you like and increase the quantity and frequency of consumption of those fab five. Like everything else that you do in this program, do it slowly and steadily at a pace you can handle.

Sometimes people don't like vegetables because their experience with them is limited to overcooked, mushy, tasteless preparations. If that is the case for you, follow a basic rule of vegetable preparation: steam them lightly for only a few minutes, maintaining a slight crunch and a bright color. As soon as they lose their brightness, they are overcooked.

Also – taste buds do change. In fact they are quite adaptable. If you are used to processed foods that have excessive quantities of sugar, salt and fat added to them (so that you will buy more), then your taste buds are out of practice at recognizing the subtler taste qualities of vegetables, fruits and other natural foods. With a more consistent intake of these nutrient dense foods, your tastes will adapt and your appreciation for them will grow in accordance.

I often hear people complain that they buy vegetables and they go bad before they use them. The key here is to use them. Cook them all at once (as above) and store in containers for use the next day. Or if your preference is to eat them raw, cut them up and store in containers for easy access. If you are noticing that some veggies have been in your fridge for a while, then search for a recipe that features those vegetables.

Keep things simple. Throughout the week when I have little time, I use the same basic preparation for all vegetables. I steam them lightly, and then add a small amount (somewhere between one teaspoon and one tablespoon) of olive oil, coconut oil or sesame oil, some fresh squeezed lemon juice, fresh ground Himalayan sea salt, fresh ground pepper and we are good to go. It's yummy, easy, and a short learning curve for those who don't know how to do fresh vegetables.

About Fruit

I know we're talking about the benefits of vegetables this week but this is as good a time as any to include a discussion of fruit as well. The reason that I didn't include it in the title as in 'fall in love with vegetables and fruit' is because most people already know that they like fruit. Understandably – it's sweet, compact and easily eaten raw. Most people eat lots of fruit but lag on the vegetable content.

It is however common for people to question whether fruit should be included in the diet when you are trying to lose weight.

I have yet to see substantial evidence in practice or theory, for weight gain by a moderate amount of fruit included on a daily basis. However, as mentioned above, it might be neutral in the sense that a variety of fruit also won't promote weight loss. So include fruit for its nutritional qualities, its alkalinity and its yumminess. But be careful not to overindulge or to use it as a substitute for vegetables.

Think about including more of the 'superfruits' (we do like our superheroes). These are the ones that score particularly high on the ORAC scale, which is one of the measures of antioxidant content. These include: all berries, especially wild blueberries, cranberries, blackberries and raspberries (also the lesser known berries: acai, chokeberries and elderberries), pomegranate, plums, and apples (especially red delicious).

Be cautious of including too much dried fruit and bananas in your diet. Dried fruit has a good amount of fibre but they are concentrated in sugar so you need to be moderate. I personally eat a couple of prunes (these score high on the antioxidant ORAC scale), dried organic cherries, or a Medjool date for dessert when I want something sweet. A little goes a long way to curb the sweet tooth. Those dried fruits are little compact sources of nutrients and sugar that win out over a baked product by a landslide, but moderation is the key. If you can't stop yourself at one to three pieces or a small handful of the little ones (raisins, blueberries, etc), I would suggest that you mostly avoid those wrinkly dried things or learn to be mindful while you eat them (see week #11, *Practice Mindful Eating*).

Bananas are also high in sugar and are certainly not needed for the potassium content because all other plant foods, including all fruits and vegetables, have an abundance of potassium.

I am not suggesting that you should never eat bananas. My suggestion is to be moderate, use a quarter or half a banana in protein shakes or in a pinch, for a quick sugar need, like when you're about to workout and you haven't eaten for a while.

Regarding juices, they contain a lot of sugar without the added benefit of a high nutrient content. In the case of fruit juice, the nutrients are depleted within approximately twenty minutes of juicing, so a commercial juice is far from ideal in nutritional value and it lacks fibre to slow down the processing of the sugar in the bloodstream. It is fine if you need a hit of fast acting sugar before or after a cardio workout or when your blood sugar has dropped too low. But that O.J. first thing in the morning would be better replaced with lemon water or fresh fruit that still has its nutrients and fibre intact. Fresh squeezed juice, drunk immediately, is, on the other hand, a rich source of nutrients in an easily digested form and could be consumed on a daily basis.

What about frozen or canned vegetables and fruit?

Canned is out but frozen is in.

In fact, in some cases, frozen can be preferable to fresh. Often frozen foods are picked fully ripe and flash frozen on site. Letting the produce ripen on the vine or in the ground increases its nutrient density and freezing it means that there will be less chemical sprays to preserve it during shipping. Having said that, local fresh food, especially organic, is still hands and shoulders above frozen.

If having it frozen means increasing your vegetable or fruit content then do it. Just watch out for any added ingredients such as fats or sugar. Get it as 100% vegetable or fruit. And remember, French fries don't count as a vegetable.

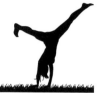

Get in Tune with Your Hunger

What you need to do

Food is such a mix of pleasure, nourishment, guilt, comfort, culture, experience and habit that it is difficult for some people to actually know whether they are eating because they are physically hungry or for some other reason. Understanding your relationship with food demands that you know why you are eating. And you can only know why you're eating by knowing what physical hunger actually feels like and noting whether or not that is taking place at any moment that you feel the urge to eat (or eat more).

This week is about paying attention to your body from the neck down to determine how hungry you really are.

Why you need to do it

Hunger and satiation signals are one way that the human body has been programmed to ensure the survival of the species. From a primitive and biological perspective, if we didn't experience hunger, we would not eat enough to ensure an adequate intake to fuel our body. And if we don't experience satiety, we may continue eating past the point of optimal functioning for our organs and tissues. It would seem from the global obesity epidemic that many have become numb to those signals. Is this purely biological? Have the dangerous ingredients in manufactured food skewed the messaging of the signals that regulate appetite? Or have we just forgotten to pay attention to those signals because food is readily available and is a quick source of pleasure?

The answer is likely a combination of both.

Researchers have established that with obesity, people can develop what is called leptin resistance. Leptin, a hormone released from the fat tissue, is one of the mechanisms that signals the brain when you are full. The leptin binds, much like a lock and key mechanism, at receptor sites within the hypothalamus of the brain. With increases in circulating leptin, you normally feel satisfied. Typically, the fatter you are, the more leptin is released to let you know that you don't need more food. However, some people will not feel that satiation despite the high levels of leptin. For them, hunger seems constant because the receptor sites are 'overworked' and no longer welcome the connection to the circulating leptin.

However, leptin resistance is more likely a symptom, not the original cause of appetite imbalance. The cause may be more closely linked to the wide-ranging effects of food manufacturing. You'll recall from week #4, *Eat Close to Nature* that manufactured foods lack the nutrients needed to generate optimal function of the body and brain. This is bad enough for the biology, but we then get hit with a double whammy. Many of those foods contain harmful additives or byproducts of processing. These chemicals wreck havoc on normal biological functions. This could include a warping of our hunger and satiation signals.

Manufacturing also means that we are also no longer in touch with the growing of our food. We have so much food available to us at any given time that our survival now depends on not eating everything that is within our reach. So in a way, we are out of practice at recognizing hunger because we rarely have an opportunity to experience it. We each need to take back control. Paying attention to your hunger signals is a simple process that yields significant rewards. When you pay attention to signals in your body and mind that tell you how hungry you are, you now have a direct line to what I would call your 'inner food guru'. This is the wisdom that you generate when you have healthy biological responses and you pay attention to the messages that your body gives you. With practice, you will no longer need to rely on someone else or a program to tell you how much or when to eat. And as you'll experience later in the program, when you learn to listen and feel for other signals in the body, that inner food guru will tell you not only when and how much, but also what foods do or don't work for your body and mind.

If you are wondering if this hunger registry contradicts my suggestion that you eat every three hours, it doesn't. It is just the next stage of refining your personal foodscape. I have clients eat every three hours right off the hop because it is common for people to go too long without eating – then they have no control, particularly at night when they are tired. Paying attention to your hunger will allow you to refine your own schedule to find your personal timing. This can change on some days and over the year might alter itself somewhat as your metabolism changes but mostly you will have a sense of the hours you can go between meals. I can actually register the hours of the day based on my stomach. I am clearly a four-hour eater. At the three and a half hour mark, I start to feel some stirring in my belly. Then within the following half hour, there is a progressive building of what I would describe as an 'emptiness'. Going longer than four and a half hours, makes me as nasty as a hunting tiger. (Or maybe it just fuels my imagination). Either way, those who know me well, know that it's not to be taken lightly if you are standing between me and my food source.

Mara is a highly intelligent woman, an executive coach, driven by self-knowledge. She had done lots of weight related programs, tracking her food, learning about nutrition, etc. She decided to work with me because she wanted to get to the core of her relationship with food. Early on in her process, I asked her to pay attention to her levels of physical hunger, to notice when she is eating or craving, if it was because of the need for fuel, or something else. She quickly discovered that she eats far more than she actually needs and that most of her call for consumption is for reasons not related at all to physical hunger. This was a revelation to her because prior to this, she had followed schedules, what others had told her, tracking calories and not on paying attention to her own body. Getting a picture on how her hunger works opened the door for her to learn what to do with the non-physical urges.

Mara's experience is common. In the next few weeks, you will delve further into reasons that you overeat, cravings and how to deal with both. However it is crucial to start with recognition of your baseline for physical hunger, so that you will know how much you actually need. You can liken this to understanding the monthly budget that you need to meet your bills and basic necessities, so that you know how much extra you have to spend, or save. Once you know the baseline amount of food that fills your physical hunger and keeps your blood sugar stable, then you can register how much extra you're eating. It is a phenomenal way to strengthen your awareness of your body. And it isn't that hard to do. All you have to do is pay attention.

How you can do it

You might think that you can't tell when you are hungry or that you never let yourself get hungry, so let's create a process to determine your level of physical hunger.

We use a tool called the 'hunger scale'. I did not create this scale. Over the years, I have seen it applied by many different eating programs, coaches and psychologists. It is used prolifically because it offers a structured way to check in with and stay aware of your physical hunger. If you look at the scale, you'll notice that zero is neutral. As you move up the scale, towards 5, you get fuller. As you move down the scale, you get hungrier. The ideal is to stay within the '2 range'.

- Higher than '2' overburdens the digestive system, depletes your energy, increases aging of the body, and encourages the storage of glucose as fat.
- Lower than '- 2' is ignoring your body's need for nourishing fuel, setting you up for blood sugar irregularities and depleting the

nutrients available to the brain to regulate the neurotransmitters, setting the stage for moodiness and emotional eating.

Most people need to eat smaller meals every two to four hours (earlier on we established 'three' as the average) in order to stay within the '2' range. Paying attention to your body's signals for hunger and satiety will tell you exactly what your ideal frequency is.

Be forgiving of yourself if you do not always stay in the '2' range. Everyone steps outside of it sometimes. When you do, it is an opportunity to pay attention to how your body feels. Note the messages of the body (see week #9, *Create a Healthy Relationship with Your Body,* for more on messaging) so that you can register the consequences of overeating or not eating frequently enough. Your motivation will get stronger the more you can register the pain of not staying within the '2' range. And remember, don't waste your energy by beating yourself up. Just notice how you feel in your body and move on so that you can do better at the next meal.

Using the scale on the next page, register how you would describe each number on the scale, in your own body. You may have other language for it than the words that have been used here.

Continue to pay attention to your hunger levels until staying within the '2' range comes as second nature for you. Or at least, you recognize when you're overeating. We'll address that in the coming weeks.

Registering Your Physical Hunger on the Hunger Scale

5	SICK
4	STUFFED
3	FULL
2	COMPLETELY SATISFIED
1	JUST SATISFIED
0	NEUTRAL
−1	HUNGER 'AWAKENS'
−2	HUNGER PANGS
−3	OVER-HUNGRY
−4	RAVENOUS
−5	EMPTY AND WEAK

Week #6

. . . .

Check Those Simple Carbs at the Door

. . .

Understand Your 'Why of Overeating'

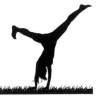

Check Those Simple
Carbs at the Door

What you need to do

If you are in a quandary about whether carbs are good or bad for you and for your weight, you're not alone. The mixed messages stemming from a variety of diets and our own desires for carbs lead to mass confusion. So let's get this clear. You need to eat the good carbs – essentially those that are complex – and get rid of, or at least minimize, the simple ones. Details about what I mean by complex and simple carbs are in the 'why you need to do this' section below. However, here's a nutshell version.

Eat vegetables (remember how beautiful those babies are), fruit, whole grains, beans and legumes. (Beans are one type of legume. Peanuts, soybeans, lentils, alfalfa and clover are some others.) Many people don't realize that all of these foods are rich in carbohydrates. They most often think of the problem carbs as the only ones there are, so all carbs get slotted as bad.

What are the problem carbs?

The sweet and starchy ones – pasta, bread, bagels, baked goods, candies, sugary foods, etc. – no surprise there. Those are also the ones that are the most tempting and that you are likely to look for in the moments of pleasure seeking. Hey, I have some good news for you. There is an appropriate time to eat these carbs. Keep reading to find out when. Also, I assure you that if you embark on the principles of protein every three hours plus lots of veggies, your physical cravings for sweet and starchy foods will diminish. I have seen it over and over again.

Rada is a successful artist, at one time a dancer. She has never had a weight issue but a reliance on sugar has been a problem for most of her 54 years. She gets deeply immersed in her work and had a tendency to ignore the needs of her body for fuel. When it came time to eat, she would grab whatever was most available – usually chocolate, candies or bread (note: these are the problem carbs). When she called me it was because she needed to prioritize her eating habits – her moods, energy and PMS were out of control and she was crying instead of dealing with her stresses in a reasonable way. Attempts at handling it by herself were proving useless. This isn't unusual because Rada was dealing with long standing habits and as human beings, we all know the challenge of changing habits. She needed simple, doable solutions that she could incorporate into her lifestyle.

We worked on the protein options that she has as an ovo-lacto vegetarian (she eats eggs and dairy but not other animal foods) and how she could ensure a three-hour eating schedule. She also incorporated vegetables, fruit, whole grains and her preferred bean varieties into her daily plan. Within one week of consistently following 'the plan' she already had more steady moods. By the fourth week, her energy was now consistently good throughout the day, her cravings were non-existent and she was thrilled that what

she thought was not possible was so much easier than she
believed it could be. By the third month, her healthy habits
were solidly in place, even for traveling, which she was doing
a lot of. The cherry on the cake (metaphorically speaking)
was that her PMS symptoms were now manageable and no
longer immobilizing.

The reality is if you don't include enough carbohydrate in your mealscape, you won't have a way of eating that is sustainable for the rest of your life. However, if you want health and lightness, you need to munch on the complex ones and check the simple ones at the door.

Why you need to do this

Complex carbohydrates have too many good things going for them to not include them in your nutrition lifestyle. Consider their benefits:

- Most efficient source of energy production for the muscles and cells and fuel for the brain.
- Complex carbs are loaded with fibre, which protects the health of digestive tract, and reduces the risk of some cancers, diabetes, heart disease and obesity.
- The combination of fibre, metabolic vitamins and minerals help to lowers cholesterol and improves detoxification capacity.
- They help to regulate protein and fat metabolism, and support muscle repair.

How then, do we define the difference between the 'problem' carbs and the 'healthy' carbs?

To answer that, we need to take a closer look at what carbs are composed of. Imagine for a moment that a carbohydrate is a train... kind of like this one:

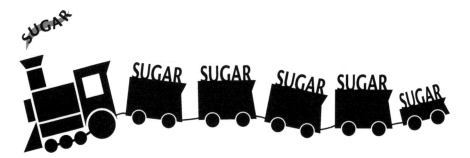

If the carbohydrate is a train, then the cars of the train are made up of sugars.

A carbohydrate is a bunch of sugar molecules, chained together that actually looks more like this (keeping in mind that this is a 2-dimensional rendition of them):

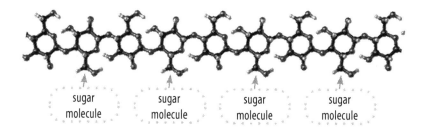

The way that we can determine which carbs are the 'problem' and which are the 'solution' is based on how many chains of sugar are bound together. This determines if they are *simple* or *complex*.

Simple carbohydrates are one or two sugars, bonded together. They are easy and quick to break apart. That means that they pass through our digestive tract and get into the blood stream quickly, providing a quick, but short-term supply of sugar.

Complex carbohydrates are three or more (sometimes, thousands of) sugars bonded together, like the one above. They take longer to break apart, and thus have a slower but steadier entry into the bloodstream.

Carbohydrates most important job is as a source of fuel for our brain and muscles.

Keeping that important job in mind, what would you guess is the better form of carbohydrate – the simple ones which get into the bloodstream quickly and then exits in the same fashion? Or the complex ones which create a slow and steady release of sugar into the bloodstream creating a consistent supply of fuel for our brain and muscle?

If you guessed 'complex', you would be spot on! And the added bonus here is that the 'complex' carbs are also the ones that are less likely to cause us to store fat.

Here is a little techno physiology about how this works.

The use of carbs as fuel for the brain and muscle, and its link to the storage or burning of fat is connected to hormone function. Two particular hormones play a key role – insulin and glucagon.

When carbs are consumed, sugar in the form of *glucose* (the simplest sugar that is used throughout the body for energy) enters the bloodstream. *Insulin* is like the bodyguard that accompanies glucose, knocking on the door of the tissue cells to tell them to let its companion glucose inside. Once glucose is inside the tissues, it will be burned as fuel or stored for later use.

The more glucose in the blood, the more insulin is needed to accompany it. A meal full of simple carbs means lots of glucose enters the bloodstream in a short period of time, stimulating a high insulin release to ensure the glucose makes it from the blood into the tissues. (Higher insulin levels have negative repercussions to your overall health as well as to your weight). The muscle tissue uses some of the glucose for an immediate fuel source and a generous portion gets shuttled to the brain, also to be used as fuel. The rest is stored in the muscle and liver for later use. Both however, have their storage limitations. Above those limitations, the remaining glucose travels to the fat cells for storage where it will stay until it needs to be broken down for fuel. However, once stored as fat, it is the 'last resort' source of energy. Muscle and liver storage will be used first. And if a continuous supply of simple carbs is consumed, without intense exercise to accompany it, the cycle of fat storage is repeated.

In simple terms here is the relationship:

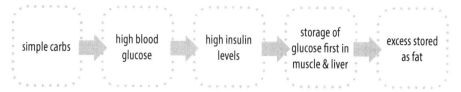

Complex carbs on the other hand, break down into glucose in a moderate and steady fashion. This releases just enough insulin to keep an adequate supply of glucose available to the tissues including the brain, both immediately and as storage for later use. However as long as you don't overeat, the complex carbs are less likely to stimulate an excess to be stored as fat.

That is a very simplified version of the role of glucose and insulin.

Now to take it a step further, insulin has an interdependent and opposing partner in this metabolic dance. That partner is *glucagon*. I referred to glucagon in the first week when talking about protein.

Like insulin, glucagon is secreted by the pancreas as a response to food consumption. But unlike insulin, which responds to carbohydrate intake, glucagon is stimulated by protein intake. Glucagon ensures that blood sugar levels don't fall too low in between meals. And most importantly for our weight loss process, glucagon is the hero in stimulating the glucose that is stored as fat to be transported from the fat cells it so that it can be burned for energy.

No food is just one macronutrient, i.e. only a carbohydrate, or only protein. All foods are a combination, to one degree or another, of carbohydrate, protein and fat. In the case of the complex carbs, particularly beans, whole grains and vegetables, they are mostly carbohydrate with a decent amount of protein (and a smaller amount of fat). Thus you automatically have a release of both insulin and glucagon when you eat those ones. This is another reason that the healthy carbohydrates (complex ones) offer a better option. The protein-carb combo supports a balance of glucagon and insulin, ensuring that glucose is favored for energy burning and not fat storage, and that stored fat will be burned between meals. Add in extra protein foods, such as eggs, fish, chicken or meat, along with the complex carbs and you better your chance of burning fat rather than storing it.

How you can do this

You may have heard of the *glycemic index* and its more useful cousin, the glycemic load. Essentially these are tools for you to determine whether a carbohydrate is a simple one or a slow, steady, complex one.

Let's talk about glycemic index first.

The glycemic index (or GI) is a measurement of how quickly a food breaks down into glucose in your body after it is ingested. Essentially then, this will tell you whether a food is going to cause a high amount of insulin release or a small amount. Remember, high insulin is more stimulating for fat storage (and will lead to related health issues such as diabetes and metabolic syndrome).

The higher the GI, the faster it breaks down and the more insulin will be released at any given time. Some examples are listed in the table below.

Note that a GI of 70 or above is considered high, in that it will break down quickly and cause a high insulin response. Between 55 and 69 is considered a medium response. And less than 55 is considered low. In an ideal world, you would eat mostly low glycemic foods, a moderate amount of medium ones and use the high ones only at the appropriate times or not at all.

Consult the chart on the next page for a look at some foods and their glycemic index

Food	GI	GL	Food	GI	GL
Sweets			**Legumes**		
Donut	108	17	Black Beans	69	7
Bran Muffin	85	15	Chick Peas	47	10
Breads			Kidney Beans	41	7
Bagel, white	103	25	Lentils	41	5
Whole Wheat	50	9	Split Peas	22	6
Baguette	136	15	**Pasta**		
Pita Bread	85	10	Linguine	65	22
Rye Bread	58	5	Macaroni	67	23
Cereals			Spaghetti	69	20
All Bran	56	12	**Snacks**		
Corn flakes	130	24	Corn Chips	103	18
Life	94	14	Jelly Beans	112	22
Special k	98	14	M&M peanuts	47	6
Grains			Peanut Butter	21	6
Quinoa	35	8	Dark Chocolate	22	7
Rolled Oats	40	2	Mars Bar	70	26
Barley	36	11	Popcorn	103	8
Brown Rice	79	18	Potato chips	77	11
White Rice	80	24	Power Bar	79	24
Fruits			Pretzels	119	16
Apple	52	6	Skittles	100	32
Banana	74	12	Snickers	78	19
Cherries	32	3	**Sugars**		
Grapefruit	36	3	Fructose	27	2
Grapes	62	7	Glucose	141	10
Oranges	60	5	Honey	78	10
Peaches	60	5	Lactose	66	5
Pears	47	4	Maltose	150	11
Pineapples	94	6	Sucrose	97	7
Plums	34	3	**Vegetables**		
Watermelon	103	4	Corn	78	9

GI Rating		GL Rating		Carrots	131	5
Rate	*Value*	*Rate*	*Value*	Peas	68	3
Low	<55	Low	<10	Potatoes	121	26
Med	56-69	Med	11-19	Sweet potatoes	87	17
High	>70	High	>20	Yam	53	13

There is a problem with the glycemic index however. It tells you how quickly a food's carbohydrate is going to be absorbed, but it doesn't take into account the amount of carbs that are actually in a reasonable portion of the food that we are likely to eat in a sitting.

This is where the *glycemic load (GL)* comes in.

The sugar in watermelon, as an example, creates a high GI. But there isn't much of that sugar in a typical serving of watermelon, so the GL is relatively low.

Since we don't normally eat one and a half pounds of carrots at a sitting or an entire large watermelon, the GL is a more useful indicator of both the quality and the quantity of carbs in a food and how it will affect insulin response.

A couple notes of caution: Neither glycemic index nor glycemic load is a gold standard of truth. Consulting a number of different resources will show some inconsistencies in the numbers. Where a food is grown and how it is prepared in cooking will play a role in the glycemic numbers. Also, the glycemic load is useful if you do not overeat. Even the low glycemic load carbohydrates can spike your insulin levels if you consume two or three servings of these foods.

The only exception to this might be green and non-starchy vegetables, which are all in the range of 1 – 3 in glycemic load. It is safe to say that no one ever got fat on leafy greens. So eat your kale, spinach, romaine lettuce and any other variety of green vegetable.

Putting this into practice

Checking where a food stands on the glycemic load is one way to determine what to eat. Having said that, you still want to maximize your nutrition by eating close to nature foods. Remember that they provide the raw materials for your body to function at its optimum. So even though M & M's and potato chips list at a fairly low glycemic load, it doesn't mean that they are in the good carb category. They are devoid of nutrition and therefore become useless, inefficient calories and potentially dangerous ones because of the chemicals and altered molecules that have been woven into the food.

In general, beans and legumes, whole grains (use brown rice cautiously and white rice isn't whole in the first place and should be avoided or at least minimized), vegetables (caution with potatoes), and fruit (not too many bananas) are excellent choices. With these foods, you get all the benefits of carbohydrates, (fibre, high vitamin and mineral content) without the negative effect of insulin spiking, which leads to fat storage.

Since protein stimulates glucagon release, eating protein and complex carbs (vegetables, fruit, beans, other legumes, whole grains) together is a surer way to stimulate fat burn.

Every meal needs to include protein. We already have that part down. At least two meals need to include an abundance of vegetables, which you now know is part of your carbohydrate intake. Fruit is an excellent source of vitamins, alkalizing minerals and antioxidants and should be eaten in moderation for long-term health.

Regarding the other complex carbs – whole grains, beans, and legumes, eat as much of as you need to have an abundance of energy throughout your daily activities and workouts. Some people will need more than others. If you have a faster metabolism and find that you feel hungry all the time and low in energy if you don't eat some starchy food such as the grains and beans, then include as much as you need to maximize your energy levels. If however, you find that you have more energy and feel clearer headed, more focused and generally healthier by having less grain in your diet, do that. This will be a bit of trial and error.

. . . .

A young professional that I'll call Nick showed up in the clinic. He is 6'5", 215 pounds and wanted to lose fat, gain muscle mass and get up to 240 lb. He had already incorporated a steady supply of weight training, five days per week. Now he wanted to take on the food component. Given some health issues that included symptoms of low energy, anxiety and lack of concentration, we started by cleaning up his diet, getting him onto close to nature foods, upping the protein and eliminating the gluten grains from his diet. Without the breads and pastas he quickly lost fat mass and gained focus, but found his energy waning during workouts. (Recall that carbs are our most efficient fuel source so they become crucial during intense workouts, whether it is cardio-based or strength training). We added in the non-gluten whole grains such as quinoa and buckwheat, more beans and lentils and more animal proteins and vegetables to accompany them. Meanwhile his trainer continued to push him harder and harder during his workouts. With a few more minor adjustments to the timing of his foods, he was up to 232 lb. of solid muscle. Nick's case is not atypical. The proper choice of quality, quantity and timing of his carbohydrates helped him get closer to his goal.

I have been talking about whole grains. Since you may not be familiar with them, let's go over what they are. I am listing them in the order of 'most nutritious to least nutritious' order. Having said that, each grain has its advantages so the list doesn't hold completely. However, if you were to eat more of the foods at the top it would be to your advantage.

- amaranth
- quinoa
- buckwheat
- steel cut or large rolled oats
- wild rice
- barley
- brown and other coloured rices
- rye, spelt, kamut, whole wheat – note that these are typically used as flours for breads and other baked products

Ideally, include more of the whole grains themselves and less of the breads. Remember that the closer it is to nature the more nutritious it will be. Having said that, if you are going to eat bread, go for the denser whole grain ones, preferably artisan breads, so that they have no chemical additives or preservatives. High quality bread needs to be frozen if you won't be eating it within four or five days. If you and your family don't consume it fast enough, store it in the freezer and take out a slice or two for toast, as you need it.

For details on how to prepare the whole grains, go to my website and click on whole grains in the resource section. There I have a graphic chart and recipes. But here's a start: I suggest that you keep this simple. I prepare most of my grains the same way. Measure your water or stock (it varies between one and a half to four parts liquid to one part grain. Bring it to a boil. Add in the measured grain with high quality sea salt (Himalayan or Celtic are good choices). When it is cooked (expanding as it absorbs the water), I add coconut or olive oil, more salt and some fresh herbs (some favorites – chives, sautéed garlic and cumin seeds, cilantro, cayenne, ginger). If you keep it simple it becomes quick to learn and easy to automate. The only other component is that most grains need to be rinsed a couple times in water before cooking. This is to get rid of the surface starch and the 'dust' that may accumulate during transport and storage. To do this, put your measured grain into a large bowl, add an ample amount of cold water. Stir it around and strain. Repeat two more times. It's then ready for cooking.

Regarding beans and legumes, I also have a chart and recipes on my site. Here is a list of the most readily available beans and legumes:

- lentils
- chickpeas
- black beans
- aduki or adzuki
- mung
- kidney
- lima
- romano

- pinto
- black-eyed peas
- split peas

The great thing about beans is that they are a good source of protein with less carb than whole grains so they have a better protein: carb ratio for fat burning. Whole grains actually have more protein per serving but they also have more carbs.

I suggest keeping your preparation of beans as simple as the grains. Once cooked, you can do essentially the same mixture as I have recommended above. One of my favorites is black beans, warmed with olive oil, lemon, salt and cayenne. When you have more time, you can do unique and more involved recipes, such as a soup or a chili. If you have less time, use canned beans. (This doesn't include baked beans due to their high sugar content). It's not perfect but we all have to find the balance between health and convenience when we have a busy schedule.

Beans can be combined with whole grains or another animal protein to up the total protein that you're getting at a meal. This is a key to cutting cravings, having steady energy and shrinking those fat cells.

Timing your carb intake

The reality is that if we are to sustain this way of eating for the rest of our lives, we cannot banish comforting carbs such as pasta and potatoes from our lives forever. So here is the trick:

If you really want your favorite starchy cuisine, **eat the simple carbs after a workout**. That way, your muscles will have just worked hard and will be in need of more glucose supply. Any extra is more likely to be stored in the muscle and liver and less likely to make its way to the fat cells.

But beware... a constant intake of high glycemic 'problem' carbs, even after workouts is more likely to slow down your weight loss than if you stick with the protein, complex carb combo pack.

If you are doing long distance cardio workouts, you can (and most likely, should) also eat the high glycemic carbs before and during your workout for a quick source of energy.

Also, given their efficient energy burn, if you do intense workouts (i.e. your heart and muscles get pushed to their max or close to) you will probably find that you have better energy during your workouts if you have a complex carb rich meal about two hours before the start of your workout session.

You might be wondering if there is another solution because you don't exercise that much and you love your comfort foods of bread, pasta and cookies. Well, I hate to be the bearer of bad news, but... too much comfort is not going to get you closer to your goals. Keep reading to find other tools to help you shift your focus to other 'sources of soothe'.

A day in the life of eating, including carbs

It can be helpful to get a picture of the ideal that you're aiming for. I am going to use the meal profile of one from my clients who has made health her top priority. She also wanted to lose weight but she knew that it wasn't going to be sustainable if she didn't get a handle on the quality of the food that she was eating.

Norma is turning fifty and has committed to being her best self at this menopausal turning point. Her personality dictates that when she decides she's going to do something, she puts everything into it. The result is that after only six months of working together she has become a model of good nutrition. Here is a fairly typical weekday for Norma. She does vary it but mostly she keeps it close to this timing and type of food because it is easy for her to repeat. She is a busy woman and automation is important for her to maintain a healthy lifestyle. On the weekend she varies it more and has more indulgences. Note the timing of her carbs on this day.

7:00 am – Breakfast:
Whey protein shake with fruit, almond milk, greens powder, flax meal and fish oil *(complex carbs – fruit, greens powder)*

10:00 am – Mid-morning snack:
Cottage cheese or Greek yogurt with fruit, nuts, and seeds *(complex carbs – some in yogurt or cottage cheese, fruit)*

12:30 pm – Lunch:
Big salad with chicken or salmon and avocado *(complex carbs – vegetables in salad)*

3:00 pm – Mid-afternoon snack:
Quinoa salad with veggies and herbs. (She makes a batch on Sunday that lasts her for three days) or mixed bean salad with veggies and herbs (she uses canned beans and makes enough for two days). *(complex carbs – quinoa, veggies, herbs, beans)*

5:00 pm – Workout:
Water

6:30 pm – Post workout:
Recovery protein shake containing only protein and carbs, banana, coconut water or juice, whey protein, berries, L-glutamine. This shake has no fat so that there is quick absorption of sugar and protein into the muscles. Fat would slow it down. *(complex carbs: bananas, berries – simple carbs: coconut water or juice)*

8:00 pm – Dinner:
Chicken, fish or meat (not the same as what she had at lunch), two colors of steamed vegetables and two types of raw vegetables on the side. She might have a little potato or sweet potato at this meal. *(complex carbs: vegetables – simpler carbs: potato, sweet potato)*

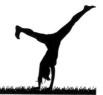

Identify Your 'Why' of Overeating

What you need to do

Last week you paid attention to what it feels like to be physically hungry, how frequently you are in need of food and how much you eat, relative to your hunger. You probably discovered that you overeat, consuming food at times that you aren't physically hungry; or you start off hungry, but keep eating past the point of your body's need. This week is about taking it to the next step. Here you can clarify what's happening at the time that your desires for food show up – when your body isn't physically hungry.

It may be helpful to categorize overeating into three different, albeit interrelated, types: stress eating, emotional eating and habitual eating. Keep in mind that there are crossovers between them – they are not mutually exclusive. An emotional eater is dealing with a particular type of stress, a stress eater has formed habits around their eating, and a habitual eater may be triggered by something in his environment that taps into emotional memories. And no one is purely one kind of eater. All of us have had experiences of each multiple times. Some of us are dealing with all of them daily.

Although figuring out why you're eating when you're not physically hungry requires the same simple process no matter what the cause, it can be helpful to recognize when you are landing in the midst of a particular type of overeating, because how you deal with it will be unique to the type.

This week then, is learning the simple process of figuring out your 'why' in any given moment. Then in future weeks you'll learn how to channel your energy to deal with it.

Why you need to do this

You want to stop the overeating but you don't know why you do it. How can you change the pattern if you are unsure of what's causing the problem in the first place? The first stage of change is recognition. Without recognition you can't prepare yourself for action. You need to be clear on what your modus operandi is around overindulgence, so that you can come up with a strategy that will support your transformation.

I referred to the various types of overeating as stress eating, emotional eating and habitual eating. Here are some details of the differences between them.

Stress Eating

Morry came to see me around six months after the death of his beloved father. Despite a busy law practice, he had been by his father's bedside everyday during his final weeks. The stress of watching his dad's deterioration and the helplessness that he felt, were, in his words, "the most challenging moments of my life." The time he had to reflect gave him insight into the powerful drive that he had to eat when he is stressed out. The extra fifty-five pounds that he carried didn't happen just because his father was dying. He realized that any form of stress – a tough situation at work, or coming home to the tireless needs of young kids after a busy day would trigger him to eat.

Stress eaters will feel the drive to eat when they are under highly charged situations that cause an overriding need to calm down, as though they've just gotten off a roller coaster.

To get a picture of how stress shows up in your body, let's imagine that you are riding your bike in downtown traffic and although you have the right of way, a bus turns towards your path, barely missing you. You narrowly escape being hit by this big honkin' vehicle and your body clearly knows it, responding by upping your heart rate, increasing your breathing and insisting on a steep rise in attention. This is your body's automated and ancient response to stress. The brain senses the threat to your survival and does what it can to mobilize you to save yourself. Lightning speed sensory input tells the brain to release a hormone called corticotropin-releasing hormone, CRH, and shortly thereafter, other hormones including epinephrine (also know as adrenaline) and cortisol. Together they offer you your best chance for survival. These chemicals catalyze signals to direct blood and energy to your muscles, causing your heart to beat faster and your metabolism to shift into high gear to produce immediate sources of fuel. Meanwhile blood flow is directed away from the more leisurely systems like digestion and immunity, which aren't needed in the immediate moment. This preparation for 'fight or flight' is designed brilliantly as a short-term adaptation. In a person with a healthy stress response, these hormones act as their own shut-off valve when enough of them reach the brain, leading your body back to a calmer state. However, in a state of continuous stress the body's responses can go awry. Long work hours, high demands on our time, pollutants in our environment, low calorie dieting, poor quality nutrition, not enough or too much exercise, disharmonious relationships, plus other types of modern day stresses can wreak havoc on our normal hormonal response. Overexposure to cortisol can result in anxiousness, depression, increases in heart rate and blood pressure, sweaty palms, excessive fatigue, foggy brain, low sex drive and an increase in appetite and cravings. Here is where stress eating comes in. What does our body want in times of increased anxiousness, low mood and tiredness? It wants to balance itself out. It wants comfort. The immediate fix is food, particularly sugar and starches, which provide quick energy. Those carbs, along with fat and salt, stimulate the production of the feel good hormones. The problem is, with excessive stress, you are faced with a continuous demand for the comfort foods and more often than not, a lack of control over your choices. Not a conducive situation for weight loss. In addition, cortisol and its effects on other hormones including insulin, promotes the storage of fat, especially around the belly. It's imperative that you are able to recognize your patterns of stress eating, so that you can strategize tools and techniques to address it.

If you discover that one of the primary reasons that you overeat is because you are a stress eater, the solution rests in a combination of good nutrition (that is laid out in this book), finding the exercise that you can be consistent with, as well as what I would term, 'creating space'. Week #8, *Nourish Your Soul* as well as week #9, *Rest and Relax to Lighten Up* will be of particular significance for you.

Emotional Eating

> *Jeannette has found that when she is facing acute stress – like when she broke up from her boyfriend of four years – she loses her appetite. She is not a stress eater. However about three weeks after the break-up, the intensity of the change calmed down and she was back to her normal appetite. That was when she started to feel lonely and was gravitating towards chocolate and ice cream. It is not an intense acute stress, but rather an aching feeling that makes her want the comfort of food.*

Technically and physiologically, there may be little difference between the stimulus for stress eating and emotional eating. Negative emotions are in themselves a form of stress, which result in a cascade of hormone release. However, when I'm referring to emotional eating, it relates more to the storage of emotional memories from the past. These emotional memories are mostly subconscious, but beneath the surface, they are powerful drivers of our behavior.

On the other hand, stress eating is more immediate. It's associated with having too much to do and having little time for reflection. There is an overwhelming sense of never-ending work and often people who stress eat, keep taking on more obligations because of addictive busyness. They seem to have an inability to slow down, although it's not really a lack of capacity. More so, it's related to a lack of practice. They rarely feel calm. The desire to eat is partly driven by the need for energy to keep going, as well as a desire for the relaxation that they can't access without substances to help them. Underlying stress eating may very well be emotional memories that caused the addictive busyness in the first place. However, I am distinguishing between them because people who would identify themselves as stress eaters need to slow down and create space, before they will be able to identify with the emotions that might be driving their behavior.

Emotional eating certainly includes moments of overwhelm and clear associations with stress. However, the more obvious experience, if one were to pay attention, is the desire to avoid negative emotions. The barrage of possibilities can show up in numerous manifestations of fear, anger, sadness, guilt, shame, loneliness, boredom, resentment, lack of purpose or frustration. In moments of negativity, what we want is 'out', a way to escape, a way to soothe ourselves. Food is a perfect foil. It is readily available, immensely comforting and socially acceptable (at least to a greater degree than the escape mode of alcohol or drugs).

If you know, or discover through this process, that you do a lot of emotional eating, don't miss out on reading and practicing the tools in week #7, *Take Charge of Your Emotions* and week #8, *Nourish Your Soul*.

Habits

Sam eats every night after dinner when he sits in front of the TV. Usually it's chips or something else salty and crunchy. When he chooses to read or play games on the internet, he doesn't think about eating. Sam is a habitual eater who is triggered by watching television.

What I have noticed about habitual eating is that it can be linked to something in your environment. A smell, a person, a place or an event can precipitate an automatic association to indulgence. Call it a 'trigger to habitual eating'. What this means is that when you encounter it, you have a subconscious drive to consume. You've done it often enough that it has formed a pathway in your brain that makes it easy to repeat. It's become a habit. If you continue to not think about it, those triggers will keep launching you into overeating.

Think of the habit as a physical pathway. You have gone down that path so many times that it's easy to walk. You can do it with your eyes closed and your attention elsewhere. In fact, that is exactly what habitual eating is like. Something triggers you and you get it in your head that you should eat and then the next thing you know, there you are, doing just that. You don't think much about it. It just happens. The pathway begins with the trigger, which prompts you to eat, and it often ends in guilt and heaviness. To deal with habitual eating, you have to alter the pathway. You need to put a roadblock in the trail to create a detour. But you can only know what roadblock will work when you are clear about what trigger(s) started you on the path in the first place. Here it is then. Awareness is the mother of transformation. You can't create real long-lasting change without 'paying attention'.

Although a habit has its basis in emotional memory, and an emotion can in itself be a trigger, I am distinguishing habitual eating as something that exists in the environment that prompts us to eat. On the other hand, stress and emotional eating are stimulated by internal discomfort.

The detective work needed to discover your personal triggers requires only a willingness to be curious about it and to pay attention. When you know what sets you up to overeat, then you can choose to mindfully break the habit.

The Six Triggers to Habitual Eating

Senses – Seeing, smelling or tasting food can be a strong trigger for many people. If looking at recipes, seeing the food in front of you, smelling it throughout the house, or tasting one little bite will cause a cascade of desire, then your senses are triggering you. For some people even the sound of chopping knives, activity in the kitchen or around the barbeque can be enough to stimulate a desire to eat.

Places – There may be particular locations that prompt you to eat: just walking into the kitchen might do it. Specific restaurants, movie theaters where you can't resist ordering popcorn and a large pop, other places of entertainment, hotel rooms, libraries (yes, the clandestine eater who gets excited by doing it in the library stacks) are all examples of places that others find provoking. If a particular location consistently causes you to crave food, it could be a signal that the place itself is a direct trigger.

People – Are there certain people that you always seem to be sharing unhealthy or large quantities of food with? Or maybe they don't eat it but influence or insist that you do. Do you have a mother or grandmother who encourages guilt for not chowing down on her edible creations? Or on the other hand, someone whom you associate with the warmth, comfort and nurturance of food that is irresistible. If being in the presence of particular people always seems to go hand in hand with excessive eating, that person is likely a trigger for you.

Times – Do you have a habit of getting that latte and cookie in the mid-afternoon whether you're hungry or not? Has an after dinner snack become a ritual taking precedence over anything else that may be happening? If there are particular times of the day that you will eat no matter what, then time might be your trigger.

Occasions – Events are one of the most common triggers because they are often associated with an abundance of food and shared indulgence. The holidays, weddings, bar mitzvahs, vacations may all cause habitual eating. This is in part because the food is abundantly available and also because of the expectation that you will eat a lot because of the occasion. Notice whether it is the presence of the food, the people, the expectation or a combination that is triggering you.

Activities – Watching television, reading, doing particular types of work, baking, or doing the bills are just a few activities that might stimulate the desire to eat. To distinguish the activity from the place in determining the trigger, notice if you would have the same desires if you were doing something else in that same location. As an example, when I'm sitting in the living room, I get triggered to eat when I'm watching TV, but not when I'm reading. So I know that it is the activity of TV watching and not the living room that is the trigger. On the other hand, if I read in the kitchen, I want to eat, but not when I read in any other room. So I know the kitchen is my trigger, not the activity of reading per se.

Weather – If dark dreary days, the joy of sunshine or any other type of weather pattern stimulates your appetite then consider it as one of your triggers. Again see if you can isolate it out from other possible catalysts such as activities and senses.

As a habitual eater, you will need to consult different weeks depending on what your triggers are but week #12, *Create a Supportive Environment* will be particularly significant.

How you can do it

I have distinguished the different types of overeating to hopefully make it easier to recognize your own patterns. However now we can simplify it down to one tool that will help you sift through that background to uncover your own idiosyncratic nature of over-consumption.

I call this tool the 'Gap of Awareness' because it's based on one fairly simple concept. If you get curious and ask yourself the right questions, the insight that follows will lead you to the right answers. The questions are easy to remember – there are only three of them. With practice you'll get faster at your responses. The questions are:

- *Am I physically hungry?*
- *If not, what is going on?*
- *What can I do about it?*

There are two 'gaps of awareness' that can be created. The easier one is the 'post-eating gap'. In this mode, you make use of the time right after eating to increase your awareness. It looks something like this:

Impulse to eat	EAT	The GAP

When you are in the 'post-eating gap', ask yourself the following questions:

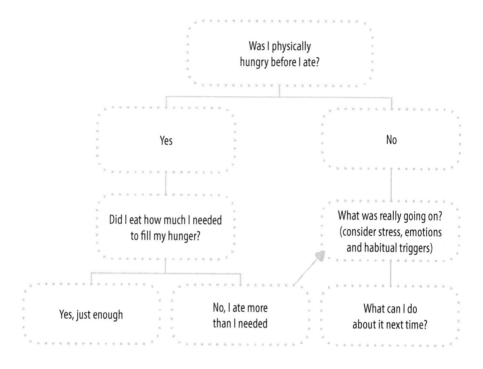

The other gap of awareness, and ultimately the one that you want to work towards practicing more often is the 'pre-eating gap'.

When you are in the pre-eating Gap, ask yourself the following questions:

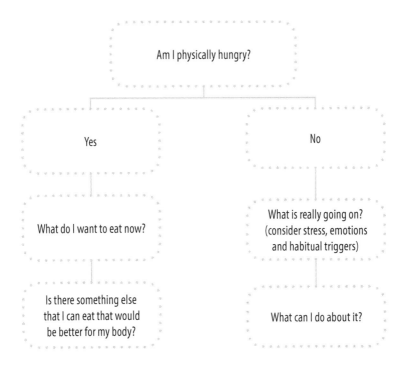

When you pay attention, you will begin to notice what triggers you to over-eat. If you feel resistant to trying this, tell yourself that you can eat if you want to – but first you need to find out what's going on. Giving yourself permission to eat, even if you're doing so for reasons other than physical need, supports you to break down the opposition to asking the questions. Inquiry is the starting point.

Remember that this week is about discovering your 'why of overeating.' As you move along in the program, you will be given tools to know what you can do about your triggers when they show up. You'll figure out which type of roadblock works best to redirect your actions and stop the automation.

Week #7

. . . .

Eat Good Fats,
Get Rid of the Bad

. . .

Take Charge of
Your Emotions

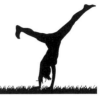

Eat Good Fats, Get Rid of the Bad

What you need to do

This week we're going to demystify fats. Like carbohydrates, they are a source of nutritional falsehoods, with the marketing machines of the food industry leading the way on deceptive info. So let's go about clarifying the importance of fats: which ones to eat and which ones to avoid. Contrary to popular belief, the right fats can help one lose fat rather than gain it.

If you recall, one of the basic principles of this program is to take on change one-step at a time and at a pace that you can handle. I hope that this is clearly engrained at this point. My wish is for you to be relaxed, to enjoy the journey and to make changes in a way that will last your lifetime. However, I am shifting out of slow lane and charging ahead in the passing lane in this case. I want you to get the importance of moving fast to take charge of your fats ASAP. Your health depends on it.

This week then is an education about fats. Then once you understand why you need to make the change, the next step is focused on helping you make the transition to health-promoting good fats and eliminating the nasty bad fats.

Why you need to do this

Unbeknownst to most people, the bad fats are some of the most dangerous foods that you can consume. They are implicated in aging, obesity, cardiovascular disease, cancer, diabetes, arthritis, autoimmune diseases and other degenerative issues. A look at the history of these altered fats shows a spike in each of these disease states as the influx of processed oils and fats infiltrated the marketplace.

Fats are like the devil and the angel, having two potential characters within the same nature. Good fats are the angels. They are needed for so many crucial functions – without them our body and mind would wither into complete malfunction. In fact, we could not stay alive without essential fats. When it comes to weight loss, they play an important role in satiation, especially when we are keeping a close reign on the carbs. They feed our feel-good hormones, which is what we often turn to sugary carbs to do. Good fats also play a role in the production and function of the reproductive steroid hormones, which will ultimately need to be balanced, speaking to the women here, to avoid the dreaded cravings that go along with PMS. As for the men, an ample supply of testosterone is needed to keep your fat burning muscles in prime form. Good fats are foundational for the balance of these hormones.

Beyond the healthy function of our hormonal system, the essential *Omega 3* and *6* fats play a further role in weight loss. They are used in the processes of metabolism. They regulate fat storage and the movement of fat out of our cells to be burned for energy. *Omega 3* and *6* along with the non-essential *Omega 9* and *short* and *medium chain saturated fats* are crucial to our vary existence and to the life of our body.

In summary, the good fats are needed for:

+ Creating fuel to burn for long-term energy
+ Insulating the body and cushioning organs
+ Producing and building new cells and maintaining the integrity of cell structure
+ Transmission of nerve impulses
+ Brain development and function

- Structure and function of eyes, hair, skin and nails, and intestinal tract
- Regulating the transport of oxygen
- Immune system support
- Hormone production
- Lowering cholesterol, prevention of cardiovascular disease
- Anti-inflammation
- Detoxification of fat soluble toxins
- The proper function of insulin, prevention of diabetes and other blood sugar issues
- Joint lubrication

Clearly, we cannot function without the good fats. We need them in ample and daily doses. However, the other side of the coin is that we are less likely to be healthy if we eat a consistent supply of bad fat.

The devil is in the nature of bad fats. These are the fats that will alter cellular metabolism and partake in degeneration. It bears repeating that heart disease, cancer, arthritis, weak immunity, mood disorders, a misfiring hormonal system, excess body fat, and diabetes, are just some of the potential issues that are linked to the consistent ingestion of bad fats.

What quality determines a bad fat?

All oils and fats are fragile, to one degree or another, to heat, oxygen and light. How much exposure one gets to each of those factors during manufacture, storage and use, will determine if it is a good or bad fat.

Let's consider manufacturing first.

Oils can be cold pressed, in which case the oil from the fruit is extracted via mechanical pressing. Olive oil, avocado oil and coconut oil are each examples of fatty fruits that have enough oil in them that they are commonly cold pressed. Many other oils, in fact most of the commercial varieties that you'll find on your grocery shelves, are chemically extracted, using hexane in the first chain of events from seed to oil. Hexane, a major constituent of gasoline, remains in trace amounts in the final oil product and is known to be carcinogenic. A lovely thought isn't it?

The delights don't end at hexane. The process further involves deodorizing in which the oils are heated to temperatures that exceed their natural tolerance, mutating them in the process. If they are going onto hydrogenation or interesterification to make them into margarines, shortenings, or fats that will be used in baked goods and confectionaries, they also include the use of heavy metals such as nickel, cobalt and aluminum and enzymes that generate altered fat molecules. They produce either a trans-fat or another equally dangerous toxic fat. The label that has been pinned on supposedly healthy margarines or other products that says 'no trans-fat' does not mean that it lacks other dangerous fats. Buzzwords float around that we either know as being good or bad but they never tell the whole story. The manufacturers of fats and oils, and most other food companies, count on you to stay uninformed so they can keep selling you their products.

Storage is another concern. Think of all those oils on the grocery shelves and in your kitchen pantry that sit there for weeks, maybe months, being exposed to light through the cheap plastic bottles. The exposure to light is further altering the structure of the fats and those altered molecules are mixing with the chemicals leaching from the plastic.

As for how we use the oils, keep in mind that some saturation makes an oil better adapted for cooking, as it is more heat tolerant. The best oils for cooking are either saturated or mono-unsaturated. The nature of polyunsaturated oils makes them more fragile to heat. They should only be added to foods after cooking.

A bit of background into the structure of fats might offer more understanding.

Fats and oils can be broken into two categories: *saturated* and *unsaturated*. The *saturated fats* will be solid at room temperature and the *unsaturated oils* will be liquid at room temperature. This is a visual indicator that you can use to distinguish between fats and oils.

Saturated fats can be further subdivided into short, medium and long chain.

And unsaturated fats can be divided into mono-unsaturated fatty acids (MUFA's) and poly-unsaturated fatty acids (PUFA's).

The PUFA's can then be divided into omega 3 and omega 6.

A flowchart of the fats might make it easier to get a picture of their groupings.

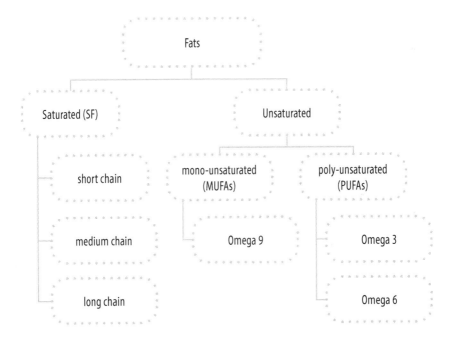

I talk more about the different types of oils, and their heat tolerance, in the next section. However as a summary, fats and oils need to go through as little processing as possible. Here is that principle again – keep it as close to nature as possible. With less processing, the oil retains more of its Vitamins A and E, lecithin, chlorophyll and the normal structure of its fatty acids. With more processing, storage, and high heat cooking, oils get destroyed and turned into toxic fats. Given that every cell membrane in the body is in part made up of fat containing molecules called phospholipids, we need to concern ourselves with the quality of the fat that we provide to those cells.

How you can do it

So what are the 'healthy' fats?

Here they are:

First the 'brilliant' ones. These are the ones that contain our much needed, and rather rare in our food chain, Omega 3's.

- **Fatty fish** – wild Alaskan or Pacific salmon, herring, anchovies, mackerel, sardines, trout, arctic char plus some others. If you don't eat fish, you should take fish oil in liquid or capsule form. Look for one that is purified of PCB's, heavy metals and dioxins either via molecular distillation or even better, Supercritical CO2 extraction, which is done at low heat without chemical solvents. The oil from fatty fish provides us with a direct source of the Omega 3 fats EPA and DHA. They are well researched for their health benefits, including brain development, mood balancing, focus and concentration, prevention of degenerative brain disorders, cardiovascular, immune, hormonal function, anti-inflammation, cancer prevention, and of course, weight loss.

- **Seeds and Nuts** – chia seed, flax seed, hemp seed, pumpkin seeds, walnuts

Eat them in their raw form to get the full benefit of the fat, fibre and other nutrients. In the case of chia and flax, they are best consumed as ground seeds. Walnuts are ideally broken open from the shell because the oil in the nut is less likely to become rancid than if they are stored outside of the shell.

In addition to the foods that are a source of Omega 3, there are some lesser known plant oils, mostly found in supplement form: borage and evening primrose oils. They contain the essential omega 6 fat called gamma-linolenic acid, or GLA for short. This fat has some excellent therapeutic benefits, particularly for menstrual issues and skin conditions. There is also some potential that may be realized in the realm of fat loss.

The oils of these brilliant fats must be in dark bottles and refrigerated after opening to protect the oil from light and heat. Do not cook with these oils.

Bare in mind that although Omega 3 and Omega 6 are the only true essential fats, in that the body cannot manufacture them from other fatty acids or carbohydrates, there is reason to keep a healthy balance of some of the short and medium-chain saturated fats and mono-unsaturated fats in your diet.

Here then are the good fats:

- Coconut and its oil
- Olives and extra virgin olive oil
- Avocado and its oil
- Other seeds and nuts – almonds, sesame seeds, sunflower seeds, hazelnuts, Brazil nuts, macadamia nuts, pecans, pistachios, organic peanuts (non-organic peanuts are high in pesticides), other nuts and seeds.

All oils of these good fats (except coconut oil) must be in dark bottles to protect the oil from light. Some also need to be refrigerated after opening to protect the oil from increases in temperature. Some can be cooked with, some cannot. Consult the fat profile chart on one of the pages to follow. To see whether it is tolerant to heat, check its smoking point. It should be at least 400 degrees to be used readily in cooking.

Now let's lay out, for all to see, the bad fats.

Trans and toxic fats – these are artificially altered fats found in any oil that has been exposed to heat, oxygen, light and/or chemicals in its manufacturing process and/or storage. These include:

- Margarine, yes even the one that is supposedly good for your heart.
- Hydrogenated and partially-hydrogenated fats
- All *mass produced oils* that are in clear bottles, colored plastic bottles and tins
- Mayonnaise and commercial salad dressings containing these poor quality fats
- Fried foods and other high heat cooking that produces smoke from the oils

- Foods that contain any of the above

Almost all oils on grocery stores shelves are of poor quality due to their manufacturing. (Look for oils in dark glass bottles from smaller specialty shops or health food stores for a greater chance of finding quality manufacturing practices.)

Plus – be cautious of:

- Barbequing
- Smoking of meats and fish
- Roasted and salted nuts
- Rancid nuts – walnuts are particularly susceptible

Some saturated fats – *commercial* meats, dairy and eggs (for more details on the commercial animal industry, go back to week #4 – *Eat Close to Nature*).

An ideal daily fat intake would look something like this:

- Eat fatty fish at least three times per week or supplement with fish oil (minimum of 650 mg of EPA/DHA daily). Research supports the daily intake of 2600 mg. of EPA/DHA combined, for fat loss
- Also, borage or evening primrose (black currant seed oil is another option but usually more expensive) for omega 6 (minimum 100 mg GLA). This is most indicated for those with skin conditions or any PMS symptoms.
- Mix one to two tablespoons of ground flax seed or chia seed into your food.
- Use extra virgin olive oil (from dark glass bottles) on salads and in low heat cooking.
- Use unrefined coconut oil or avocado oil for cooking at moderate to higher heat.
- Eat one-quarter to one-half an avocado and a small mixture of raw nuts and seeds – as an example, ten almonds, three walnuts from

the shell, two brazil nuts, two tablespoons of pumpkin, sunflower, hemp or sesame seeds.

- Buy oils that are in dark glass bottles, as they are all fragile to light (coconut oil is the exception).

- Eat only lean cuts of pasture-raised or wild meats, fowl, and the eggs and dairy from these animals.

- Avoid all processed foods in general but especially the ones with processed fat.

The poly-unsaturated oils should be in dark, glass bottles to protect them from the light and the leaching of chemicals from plastic. They should be kept in the fridge when not in use. They should not be heated, and should be capped quickly after use to protect them from oxygen.

The mono-unsaturated oils should also be in dark glass bottles (unless they are going to be used within weeks of bottling) but they don't need to be kept in the fridge and some can be used for cooking. Check the fat profiles in the chart to follow for the oils that have the highest smoke points. These are the ones that are most tolerant to heating.

How much fat should you get each day?

If you follow the ideal recommendations above and choose a little bit of fat at each meal, you will be getting what you need.

However when talking about quantity, approximately 30% of caloric intake should be good quality fat.

If you are into numbers, like thinking in calories, and want to work out a formula, consider this:

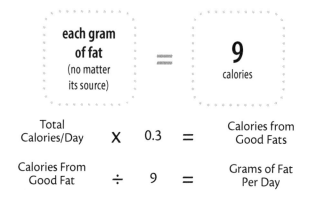

| Total Calories/Day | X | 0.3 | = | Calories from Good Fats |
| Calories From Good Fat | ÷ | 9 | = | Grams of Fat Per Day |

An example:

For an 1800 calorie diet, the ideal amount of fat (at 30%) would be:

| 1800 Total Calories/Day | X | 0.3 | = | 540 kcal should be generated from good fats |
| 540 kcal | ÷ | 9 | = | 60 grams of good fat per day |

We need an equal amount of saturated, mono-unsaturated, and poly-un-saturated fats in our body in a ratio of 1:1:1. Therefore in the example above you would need about 20 grams of each per day.

Here is a chart that summarizes good sources of each.

Good sources of the Various Fats and Oils

Saturated Fats	Mono-Unsaturated	Omega 3 Poly-Unsaturated	Omega 6 Poly-Unsaturated
• Coconut and oil • Eggs (from naturally raised fowl) • Organic milk, cheese, butter • Meat (lean cuts from grass-fed, free grazing animals)	• Olive oil, olives • Almonds and oil • Avocado and oil • Hazelnuts and oil • Brazil nuts • Macadamia nuts/oil • Pecans • Peanuts (organic only) • Pistachios • Sunflower seeds/oil • Other nuts and seeds	• Fish oil, cod liver oil • Fatty fish: salmon, mackerel, herring, sardines, anchovies, plus • Flaxseeds and oil • Chia seeds • Hemp seeds and oil • Dark leafy greens • Krill oil • Phytoplankton	• Evening primrose oil • Borage oil • Black currant seed oil • Hemp seeds and oil • Sesame seeds and oil • Walnuts and oil • Pumpkin seeds/oil • Other nuts and seeds

In actuality, no fat or oil is completely one type. All fats have some saturated fat in them and variant amounts of mono and poly. Check the chart on the next page to see the breakdown plus the heat tolerance of each fat. Remember that you want an oil to be tolerant to at least 400 degrees to use it freely in cooking. If I didn't mention a high heat tolerant oil as a good choice for cooking, it is because it is either hexane extracted, not readily available or both. Grapeseed oil is an example of one that is hexane extracted. Macadamia nut oil is great for high heat and might be found cold-pressed in gourmet food stores but it is not easy to find.

Keep in mind as you review the chart of fat profiles, that the nut or seed in its whole form might have a slightly different fat profile than the oil itself. As well, oils will vary in their fatty acid profile dependent on growing conditions and oil production. Smoke points can vary based on how refined the oil is, frequency of use, quality of manufacturing and purity of oil.

Chart of Fat Profiles

OIL *	% SF	% MUFA OMEGA 9	% PUFA OMEGA 6	OMEGA 3	SMOKE PT. (°F) **
Almond	7	65	28	0	430
Apricot Kernel	6	63	31	0	495
Avocado	17	65	18	0	520
Beef Tallow	55	40	5	0	400
Black Currant	8	12	80	0	225
Borage	14	22	60	0	225
Butter	65	32	1	1	350
Canola	12	24	54	10	350
Cashew	18	70	6	0	390
Chia/Salba	10	6	20	64	225
Chicken Fat	31	49	20	0	375
Coconut	91	8	1	0	450
Corn	13	27	59	1	320
Duck/Goose Fat	35	52	13	0	375
Evening Primrose	10	9	81	0	225
Fish	25	0	0	75	235
Flax Seed	9	18	16	57	225
Grape Seed	9	15	76	0	400
Hazelnut	10	75	15	0	425
Hemp Seed	10	15	54	21	225 -300
Lard	40	48	12	0	365
Macadamia	12	84	2	2	400-450
Olive	15	72	12	1	250-375
Palm	51	39	10	0	450
Palm Kernel	85	13	2	0	450
Peanut	18	48	34	0	275-300
Pecan	8	66	26	0	450
Pistachio	15	54	31	0	325-350
Pumpkin Seed	17	20	60	3	250
Rice Bran	26	46	27	1	500
Safflower	8	14	78	0	300
Sesame	15	40	45	0	250-300
Soybean	15	24	56	5	300
Sunflower	12	19	69	0	300
Walnut	9	28	58	5	320
Wheat Germ	17	22	53	8	225

Take Charge of Your Emotions

What you need to do

If you have struggled with your weight, you likely have your own personal brand of emotional eating. Let's call it an 'emotional food imprint' – it's a pattern that a person runs over and over again to avoid what they don't feel they can handle. It may be boredom, the avoidance of work, the intensity of anger, the sadness of being alone, the frustration of being misunderstood, or some other personal discomfort. Those who relate to food in a dysfunctional way, have some emotion(s) that they don't know how to take charge of. Whether we are aware of it or not, food becomes one way that we tone down the intensity of the feelings we're having.

. . . .

I remember the moment that I opened the fridge and had an 'ah ha' moment, seeing myself clearly lodged in avoidance mode. Prior to making my way to the fridge, I had been sitting in front of my computer for twenty minutes – I was due to deliver an overview for my first website. I was still stuck on trying to find the words for the first paragraph of the homepage. Writing has never come easy for me, and writing copy is the hardest. I was feeling overwhelmed and all I wanted was to do something else. This wasn't a new feeling. In fact, I would often get overwhelmed in the early stages of my business. As often as I would have this feeling, I would be at the fridge looking for food. Eating made me temporarily forget that I had anything else to do. The moment that I got that I wasn't really hungry, that I was just replaying a pattern, I closed the fridge and went back to my writing. Four websites later, I still don't like doing copywriting but I no longer eat to avoid it.

By eating, we can temporarily 'turn off and tune out' whatever is bothering us. For a moment or two in time, we can exchange the inner turmoil for the immediate pleasure of those crunchy kettle chips or that soft creamy ice cream sundae.

There is a problem with this though. We all know it.

The problem is that the emotion doesn't go away because we eat. We might have shoved it down sufficiently for a moment in time. But it will rear its head once again. Next time, chances are we will repeat the 'emotional food imprint' and eat again. More eating. More fat. More self-aversion. And the cycle continues.

This week then, is focused on taking charge of your emotions so they don't take charge of you. It is about understanding why you need to stop resisting what you're feeling and start (or continue) practicing the tools that support you to deal with the emotions as they come up.

Why you need to do it

If you function well without paying too much attention to your feelings, you may wonder what's the point. It's the nature of some people to get along in life mostly by staying productive, by exercising off their stress, by focusing their attention outside of themselves and on what they consider to be more important than their own emotions. If your body and mind are as you wish them to be, if you feel fulfilled, relatively peaceful and satisfied, then all the power to you. You have figured out a way of 'doing life' that works for you.

However, let's assume that you are reading this book and interested in this chapter, because you are not living the life that you ideally would like – there is a 'tuning out' somewhere – either in how you relate to food, to your body, to yourself, to others and it's being reflected in the life around you. Ignoring this 'tune out' will keep you stuck in your patterns. You need to get connected to whatever is disconnected. If you don't fully accept who you are, then you need to go through a process to free yourself.

Susan is an executive coach in her forties, who revealed early on that she had been sexually abused when she was a child. She had done a lot of therapy to get to the point where she could speak easily about it. However she hadn't yet made the link between her childhood experience and her relationship with food. Her 'emotional food imprint' is that whenever she was feeling insecure, or vulnerable, she would eat. Food helped her feel safe. Her fat had also become a protection. She believed that if she were fat, no one would want her sexually.

Barnard is determined to have an exciting life. He loves adventure. He also admitted to the tumultuousness in his relationships and his attraction to emotional drama. He overeats when he's bored. He associates boredom with an ordinary, mediocre life. Food helps him escape from that possibility, at least temporarily.

Maria eats whenever she's happy – it's the way she chooses to celebrate. She comes from a large Italian family and there are many opportunities to celebrate with food. In fact, even if she isn't celebrating, food holds an association of happiness for Maria.

Sarah doesn't yet have clear boundaries for herself. She often finds herself saying yes to friends and co-workers when what she needs to do is think it through to see if it feels right for her to say yes. She gets angry as a result. She used to think it was others that she was angry at for putting her in that position. She felt like she had no power or control over her life. Food temporarily gave back her power. She chose what and when she ate, and no one could stop her from that.

Each of these people has their own version of an 'emotional food imprint'. They, like all of us who emotionally eat, need to become aware of what that pattern is. Last week, I introduced you to the 'gap of awareness.' The GAP gives you the opportunity to use your moments of overeating as a way to clarify what happening internally. It's like shining a light on the present moment. It's a shot of recognition. When you can see what you're really feeling, then you have options for changing what isn't working for you.

People who are practiced at emotional self-expression exude more confidence and self-respect. They are more in control. As a result, their 'emotional food imprint' starts to change. They no longer feel the impulse to eat merely to disconnect from their emotions. They consciously choose when, what, and how much they need to eat. Beyond their relationship with food, there is a greater sense of freedom and an openness of heart. It is easier to love unconditionally, to believe in their lovability, and to consistently be in a place of acceptance. This would be enough reward, but attunement with our emotions offers even more. It means higher intelligence, stronger immunity, better digestive health, and a far greater resiliency in managing stress.

The Institute of HeartMath (IHM), which focuses its research, training and tools on the health of the heart, offers some great insight into the value of being in charge of our emotions. *Science of The Heart: Exploring the Role of the Heart in Human Performance* is IHM's overview of their research. I like this succinct reference from their text regarding the importance of emotional input to our intelligence. "Neurologist Antonio Damasio stresses the rationality of emotion in his book, *Descartes' Error*, where he emphasizes the importance of emotions in decision-making. He points out that patients with brain damage in the areas of the brain that integrate the emotional and cognitive systems, can no longer effectively function in the day-to-day world, even though their mental abilities are perfectly normal."

This is supported by the research behind emotional intelligence (EI). People who have a higher level of EI as opposed to IQ have greater success in the world.

A reference to a study done on emotions and immunity, concluded: "Heart-focused, sincere, positive feeling states boost the immune system, while negative emotions may suppress the immune response for up to six hours following the emotional experience."

This makes sense since emotions directly affect the autonomic nervous system (ANS). The ANS either directly or indirectly regulates activity in the immune system, the heart, muscles, blood vessels, digestive tract, hormone-releasing glands, and other body parts. The effect of emotions extends beyond our head. Our entire body is impacted by emotional patterns.

The old paradigm that the emotions remain confined to the brain is narrow thinking. Clearly there is a body-wide response to emotional experiences. But what is amazing is that science is now supporting what many of us who have worked with emotional healing have suspected for a long time: that it is not just the response to a present emotional experience that is felt in the body, but also that unconscious emotional memories are stored throughout the cells and tissues of our entire structure. As a result we repeat patterns due to neural and hormonal pathways that have been well entrenched in our nervous system.

Research from the 1980's revealed that emotions are neuropeptides, a type of protein molecule. They have receptor sites located across parts of the brain that process emotions, as well as organ systems through the rest of the body. What this means is that the molecules of emotion travel beyond the brain to store, like a lock and key mechanism on the cells of the organs. There is a part of the emotional brain called the amygdala that plays a central role in this process. This little almond-shaped part of the brain works in concert with our naturally occurring stress hormones to catalyze unconscious emotional memories, the memories that we don't recall. Pump up the stress, the more the amygdala tells the other parts of the brain that it is important to store this experience in the memory banks. The amygdala has a network of connections throughout the brain, and this network sends its emotional neuropeptides to various regions of the body. The more times we repeat an emotion, the more receptor sites develop to receive the emotional molecule. So even though that emotion may not be accessible to our conscious mind, our body knows it.

My friend Joan is a long-time practitioner and teacher of yoga. She was relaying a story to me about being in a posture where she is sitting with her legs together, aligned in front of her. The stretch involves bending at the hips while keeping the back straight, allowing the upper body to fold towards the legs. Initially she was stuck in an almost upright position but as she stayed in the posture, strong emotions welled up and she started weeping. Progressively, as powerful feelings flowed, she was able to bend towards the legs until she was almost folded in half. Joan said that she had no idea what she was weeping about but the movement triggered something in her body. The initial resistance in her hips seemed to be a reflection of some emotional resistance that she wasn't conscious of, but her body was.

Candace Pert, PhD, neuroscientist and author of the book, *Molecules of Emotion,* talks about how unexpressed emotions are literally lodged lower in the body. Signals from the amygdala generate chemicals and impulses that function to keep the emotion in the body and in the cells where they are stored. As a result we will consistently experience the same emotions over and over again until we do the work to move the emotion out of the cells and through the nervous system. Her theory for healing emotion is that these stored molecules must be expressed through the body and then travel up the spinal cord to be brought into awareness. This is easier said than done because there is a natural need to resist the emotion. This resistance is coming from the neocortex of the brain. Quoting from Dr. Pert, "the cortex resistance is an attempt to prevent overload. It's stingy about what information is allowed up into the cortex. It's always a struggle in the body. The real, true emotions that need to be expressed are in the body, trying to move up and be expressed and thereby integrated. That's why I believe psychoanalysis in a vacuum doesn't work. You are spending all your time in your cortex, rather than in your body. You are adding to the resistance."

I spent twelve years focused on my own emotional healing. My personal experience supports Dr. Pert's theory. There are some emotions that just can't be dealt with through talk therapy or any technique that does not involve body release. The physiological networks are too strong. Professionally, I have witnessed the same. When I have presented my ideas in interactive group workshops using expressive movement and sound (see BLMS to follow), the feedback has been profound. One man from Holland came up to me after a session to say that for all of his adult life, he had been looking for a way to express his emotions and he finally found a method in what we had just done. Standing ovations at the end of these highly interactive workshops are routine. I share this with you only to give you a sense of the power that free expression through the body can have for people, as long as they are open and willing to experience it. There are some emotional situations that can be dealt with through verbal expression or various cognitive techniques. But if an emotion has a stronghold in your memory banks, those circuits cannot be disrupted unless you get into your body to change them. This is particularly true if you experienced trauma in your childhood when you were in a developmentally vulnerable stage. Call it healing the old wounds, freeing the inner child, or releasing the pain body. I have heard many references to it. The important point is that the deeper the pain, the more it will depend on you moving it through your body. The mind just can't handle this job alone.

How you can do it

The thing to keep in mind is that it is not your feelings that will hurt you. It is the resistance to them that will. If you continue to resist, the pattern will persist. As a result, you will stay heavy – in mind, heart and body.

Susan, who I mentioned above, was a gift of a client for me. As a woman who needed to lose about seventy-five pounds and had a history of sexual abuse, it took courage for her to look at her emotional food imprint. But as a person who places a high value on self-growth, she was willing. She wanted to develop a love for her body, for its own sake, and also to attract a partner. She chose to use free dance, writing and visual art to express her pain. We etched out a nutrition lifestyle that worked for her and she used her indulgent times, the times that she veered off the path, as an opportunity for reflection. She would journal what she was feeling. She put on music to dance to. She did walking meditations in nature. She went to yoga classes. She talked about how she would cry so deeply that she felt like she was crying for the whole world. Despite experiencing the pain of her past, she described how rich her inner life was becoming. Rather than dreading the binge eating that she used to do, she looked forward to her time alone. She continued journaling as a way to expose the dark hidden crevices to the light. She was feeling lighter, freer. She continued to use her emotions as an exploration into what was going on for her. Slowly and steadily over a period of one year, Susan lost forty pounds. She was excited about her journey. She knew that she was on a path that would change her life. We concluded our relationship but stayed in touch periodically over the years. Five years later she had lost the seventy-five pounds and was living with a man that she claimed was the love of her life. Working with Susan was an honour, because I was given the gift of witnessing a person develop a deeper level of wisdom, peace, self respect and confidence. It is an amazing process to behold. I encourage you to take your own journey. It does take courage and openness, but it will be worth the effort.

Handling our emotions in a healthy way means having tools to deal with those emotions. Few will enter into the dragon's den of feelings if they think they will be stuck there, in that sometimes dark, intense place. We need to know that there are maps to help us make our way through to the other side where calm resides. Knowing that we have a way through, helps extinguish our brain's resistance to facing the emotion.

Let's dissect emotions so that you can understand what you are experiencing and then choose how to deal with it.

Every emotion has two parts:

1. The Story

This is experienced in the mind. It is composed of beliefs, perceptions, and thoughts. It will keep you circling around and around, questioning, obsessing, and judging. Words you might use when you are in your story are angry, frustrated, pissed off, sad, lonely, blame, 'he did this...', 'then she said...', etc.

Sarah, who had trouble with her boundaries used to express her story something like this "Jack always asks me to cover for him when his caseload gets too heavy. He expects me to work weekends when he chooses to take off to go sailing. He pisses me off. I can't believe he can be so arrogant to assume that my time is less important than his."

2. The Sensation

This is experienced in your body. It is composed of a feeling and might have visual and auditory sensations to it as well. This is the route to being present with your emotion and being able to move it through to recognize and release it. Ways of describing the sensation might be 'a knot in my stomach', 'tightness in my chest', 'it feels red hot', 'a lump in throat', 'a grey emptiness in my belly', etc.

When I directed Sarah to her body and the sensation that she was experiencing when she talked about Jack, she described "heat that ran from her belly to her throat, with a pulsing around the heart area."

Notice the difference in the quality of the language between the story and the sensation.

Being able to call an emotion for what it is, such as I am angry or sad, or lonely is beneficial, maybe even necessary. But once it is identified, it is best dealt with by experiencing it as a sensation. Otherwise that resistance that the brain has, to allowing stored emotion to move into conscious awareness, will be hard to overcome.

Once you have the sensation, then it is time to apply one or more tools to work through it. Some ideas for this are listed below. Before you get going, I want you to know a bit about the outcome. When you have cleared an emotion via your body, a couple things are probable: You will feel calmer. It is also possible that you won't be able to think about the initial source of the discomfort. In other words the story won't exist anymore, other than as a memory of having had it in the past. Peacefulness will often accompany the calm and you might feel the need to sleep. Emotional release requires energy, sometimes a lot of it. So give yourself some space and know that your tiredness is well earned.

Build an emotional release toolbox

Consider the carpenter or the handyman who routinely keeps his toolbox with him to have access to the tools needed for the work at hand. Without those tools, the job just can't get done. Preparation is required to ensure that the tools are readily available to increase efficiency and effectiveness. Experience is also needed to know how and when to use each particular tool.

We can use the handyman's toolbox as a metaphor for our emotional toolbox. The idea is to have what you need in one place (in your mind) to perform the work of emotional release as it comes up. Understanding what tools you have at your disposal is the first order of business. But it is only through experimentation, practice and experience that you will learn what works well for you. Openness to try new things is crucial for anyone who does not have a well-honed and successful practice for dealing with their emotions.

Let's start with identifying what you already have in place that you can throw into your toolbox.

Think back to times that you have dealt successfully with your emotions, stepping away from the circumstance feeling more positive and calmer than when you started.

What tools did you use during those times?

Metaphorically, you can throw these tools into your toolbox. Practically, what you can do is to write them down.

If you know that you need more resources than what you already have, consider the following options.

Emotional release tools

Talk with a trusted friend, family member, coach, councilor or therapist – Choose someone who you know will not judge, yet will aid you to see a broader perspective. Stay away from those who drain your energy or who like to dwell in your pain with you. Let that person know not only what you are experiencing but also what you would like to see as an outcome, in other words, *how you would like to be with this situation*?

Journal your thoughts and feelings – Set an intention for your journaling. (See the principles to follow). Once that is done, let your feelings go. If you do not feel safe to do so, as someone might find it and read it, then remind yourself that you can shred or burn your writing right after. The important thing is to express yourself fully. A good exercise for journaling is 'morning pages' that Julia Cameron refers to in her book *The Artist's Way*. This is a practice that includes twenty minutes each morning (or at another pre-ferred time of the day) when you write freely without editing. Keep your pen to paper or fingers to computer and just write whatever free associations come to mind.

Get physical – Go for a walk, to the gym, for a swim, ride your bike, dance to your favorite music, roll around on the floor. Any movement will do. The practice here is to get used to free movement as opposed to just exercise. The distinction was made in week #4, *Find the Exercise that is Right for You*. Free movement leaves room for anything that might happen in your living room, backyard, with your kids or pets, or while you're making dinner. It gives you access to your body at any point rather than just when you can get to the gym. (Although the gym is good too.) Do whatever turns you on and do it as you need it.

Yoga – This 'exercise' deserves its own mention because it encourages slowing down and creating a deeper connection with the body, giving room for release to happen. Joan's story that I mentioned above is an example of what often happens in a consistent practice of yoga. In the yogic lifestyle, the physical postures are the preparation for the mind to find stillness in meditation. The idea is that stress is released through the body so you can find peacefulness and can reflect on a higher state of awareness.

Get out into nature – Nature is calming. Unlike us, nature does not have an ability to be introspective, so there is no questioning or judgment about itself. It is perfect as it is. This allows us to share in that non-judgmental perfection. Use it as a place to reflect and release, remembering the basic principles that I have listed on the following pages.

Paint, draw, or do some work with your hands – The mind can only focus fully on one thought at a time, so putting your energy into some kind of creative project with your hands is a great way to both dissipate the emotion and reflect on it. Creativity encourages exploration, curiosity, and problem solving. It is a natural accompaniment to generate positive emotions and positive outcomes to discomforting emotions. Keep your intention about the outcome clear so that your creative work is drawn towards reflection. That shifts it from avoidance to clearing.

Emotional Freedom Technique – EFT, for short, is a type of self-help acupuncture. The creator of the technique, Gary Craig, offers the basic process for free at his site, www.garythink.com. There, you can download the manual and watch videos that demonstrate how to do it. It is a simple process and my experience is that it can be powerful, either on its own, or used along with some of the other tools listed here.

HeartMath or other body-based techniques – There are many modalities that are focused on emotional healing. If you are intuitively drawn to one, give it a try. You may find that it is powerful for you, offering a strong catalyst for your healing. Or you may need to experiment with many to see how each benefits you. It helps to find experienced practitioners for the techniques that you choose.

Listening to Music – Music, chosen to suit your mood, next to exercise, is one of the fastest ways to de-stress. It can also be used as a catalyst to release painful feelings. The key is to choose music that is compelling for you at the time and to actually listen to it, rather than just have it as background sound. Best to put your headphones on and let it take you deeper into its recesses so that you can find common ground.

BLMS (Breath, Light, Movement, Sound) – This is my baby – the technique that I teach to most of my female clients. Not that men can't do it. They can. It's just that most men are not as inclined to this style of clearing – they gravitate more to concrete actions like exercise, walks in nature and talking to another trusted person or to a professional. Women are particularly receptive to using their body to clear their emotions. I love this technique and find it to be singularly the most powerful way to ground a person in their body, to give them real release and to help them find a sense of calm and clarity. Start with breath. Then progress through the steps, as your body needs to. Only minutes of this can clear your emotion and give clarity to your situation. You can read more about how to do BLMS to follow. Keep in mind however, that it is only by experiencing it and practicing it that it will have any power for you.

There are some principles to keep in mind, to make emotional release powerful:

Get the emotions out of your head and into expression – Whether it is through movement, your voice, your pen, paints, or whatever tool you choose to use, this principle is foundational. It is a reminder to get past your story and into the sensation so that you can override the resistance that the brain has to receiving the emotional stimulus.

Be clear about your intention – What do you want the outcome to be? If it is to create change, then think about what you want that change to be and go into the process with that in mind. There is a big difference in how you approach it if you are going into your emotions with no intention, or the intention just to let off some steam, and if you go in with the intention for change.

As I was going through my own period of conscious emotional release, I would consistently run into the pattern of resentment and anger towards my partner at the time. In moments of angst, he was an easy target to blame. I knew rationally that he was (metaphorically) like a mirror, holding up a reflection for me to see something about myself. So at the start of any session of journaling or free movement, I

set an intention 'to find and create unconditional love,' or
'to be at peace with this situation'. What came out of my
healing sessions was just that – a more profound acceptance
of myself and my own needs and an easier detachment from
his choices.

You need to feel safe – Safety rules. Whatever environment you are in, it must feel safe for you, or you will not feel the freedom to fully express yourself. Your sub-conscious mind will be occupied with thoughts of protection. If there is no one that you feel safe to do this with, do it in the confines of your own space and set it up as a safe, comforting and sacred place to be.

If you cannot deal fully with an emotion at the time it comes up, make a commitment to deal with it as soon as you can – That might mean when you get home that evening, when you have more free time on the weekend, or when you are in the company of your support person(s). The key is to not ignore them. If emotional awareness had seven deadly sins associated with it, 'ignoring' would be high on the list. Breaking patterns that no longer serve you requires you to be diligent in dealing with your emotional issues. If you don't – the emotional food imprint will continue, whether you are conscious of it or not.

Summarizing How to Address Your Emotions

- Name them. *What emotion am I experiencing right now?*
- Feel them. *How is it showing up in my body?*
- Deal with them. *Use the tools that you have in your toolbox or others that you adopt.*

BLMS – Breath, Light, Movement, Sound

This is a technique that I created from years of practice and teaching of free movement, along with sounding, the visual arts, and conscious breathing. Although I started dancing for the pure expression of what I was experiencing musically, the process of this movement seemed to catalyze and release deep-seated emotion, bringing it to the surface and also providing me with a tool to express it. In passing on what I have learned, it became clear that others also found power in this technique.

Here are the written directions to practicing BLMS. However, the power of it can only be understood by experiencing it.

1. Name your emotion. *Ex: I am feeling angry.*

2. Find it in your body. How does it show up? Where is it? What does it feel like? *Ex: It is showing up as tightness in my shoulders and neck. It feels like it is compressing my heart area. Or, it feels like nervousness in my stomach – twitching and hot.*

3. Breathe into it. Breathe deeply, directing your breath to the area. Continue to do this until the feeling changes in some way or completely dissipates.

4. If the breathing does not calm your body and mind completely, shine an imaginary light into the area where you are still experiencing a sensation. Follow the light in and see how it looks in there. Keep breathing and shining the light and watch to see if and how the sensation changes. Note that this component works for some people but not others. If it doesn't do anything for you, move to step #6.

5. Check in with the initial emotional experience to see if it still holds any discomfort for you. If it doesn't, and you feel calm, you can stop here. If it does, repeat the process or move onto the next step.

6. If breath and light don't shift you into a state of calm, then use movement. Stand up, close your eyes, and ground your feet. Let your body guide your movement. However your body feels like moving, follow it. This might be just a simple rocking motion or you may be driven to flailing arms and vigorous leaping, or something else. Whatever your body wants, go for it without judgment. Keep breathing throughout, exhaling through your mouth. Use music if you feel inclined. Dance lightly or wildly. Trust your body to guide you in how it wants to move.

7. Let out any sound that needs to be expressed. This can start with verbal exhales. However don't stop there if there is any impulse to make louder and/or creative sounds. Sounding can be the final catalyst for deeply stored and painful emotions.

8. Check in with the emotional experience that catalyzed this process. You will know that you have cleared it when you either feel completely calm, or you can't think about it at all. If there is any residue remaining, repeat the process or continue moving and sounding more vigorously.

Week #8

. . . .

Think 90/10 for Sustainability

. . .

Nourish Your Soul

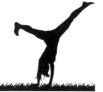

Think 90/10 for Sustainability

What you need to do

Eat well (by the principles set out in this program) 90% of the time and your body will handle the indulgences that you choose 10% of the time. This principle is one more way that you will prep yourself for the rest of your life. It gives you permission to veer outside your regular routine of eating, into the pleasurable sins of apple pies, cheesecake, bagels with cream cheese, triple cream brie or whatever other delights you choose. This is a perspective shift away from the doldrums of constant calorie counting into the specifics of how much you can indulge and what you should choose to indulge in.

Why you need to do this

If you don't give yourself room for your favorite treats, then you are bound to long-term failure. I have not met a single human being who didn't have their personal food and drink pleasures of choice. I routinely ask those I socialize with, "if you were stranded on a desert island for the rest of your life, what five foods would you bring with you, if nutrition was not a concern?" Invariably at least two or three of everyone's choices are high in fat and sugar or fat and salt. It's understandable because our brains are programmed to look for foods that offer satisfaction. It is the human, actually the mammalian, genetic drive for pleasure. And what offers more gratification in the food realm than sugar and fat, salt and fat or all three? It appears that in us mammals, nothing provides more satisfaction, unless you prefer to bypass food and go for other addictive substances, such as alcohol, cocaine, or another drug. In the book *The End of Overeating*, Dr. David Kessler outlines research by Sara Ward, PhD that was published in 2005. Ward used the meal replacement, Ensure, which is high in both sugar and fat to test how much work mice are willing to do in order to earn the food reward. Ward states, "the breaking point at which the animals would no longer work for the reward, is slightly lower that the breaking point for cocaine. Animals are willing to work almost as hard to get either one."

So, fellow human beings, let us not underestimate the power of food for pleasure. To deny it, is to risk the eventual pitfalls of the naiveté.

Being at your ideal weight is dependent on you being realistic to what you can and will give up and being clear that there will be times when you will choose to indulge. People who live in a healthy and light body are practiced at their excesses. They have control mechanisms in place. They question whether a particular extravagance is worth it or not.

Over time, as you learn to pay closer attention to your body, you'll understand your limits and become confident in your ability to recover when you push past them. This practice does depend on the foundation of a mostly nutritious diet, thus the 90% of 90/10. Without a high nutrient content, your brain and body won't be able to deal with the 'food drug' of choice. The biological factors that stimulate your addictions will ultimately win out.

The times that are commonly indulgent, such as the holidays, family gatherings or some other social event, are when you're likely to find yourself being challenged by a shift away from routine. There are constant temptations during these times when there are vast quantities of yummy food. There's nothing wrong with allowing yourself a little more lusciousness than what exists in your regular day-to-day mealscape. However you need to prepare yourself for this. Consider it a kind of 'indulgence training.' You can liken it to a marathon. If you were to enter one without conditioning, you would be hard-pressed to make it close to the finish line. When faced with a marathon of holiday parties or wedding celebrations, you're unlikely to make it to the end of the festivities in a healthy and light condition if you don't prepare yourself. You'll need to break away from the "all-or-nothing syndrome" that has always been one of the great downfalls of typical diets and weight loss programs. Plan your indulgences, figure out your limitations and get to know the diet vices that you have no control over. This will teach you to find a rhythm to your eating that works to keep you in balance. The principle of 90/10 won't be perfect for everyone all of the time, but it's a great starting point. It offers you a practical perspective on how many times in a week you can treat yourself, so that you are picking what's really worth it, and what you can more readily give up.

How you can do it

Let's do some calculations:

If you are awake for sixteen hours per day and eat five meals (we're counting snacks as a meal) in that time, you would be eating thirty-five meals per week.

$$35 \quad \text{X} \quad 0.10 \quad = \quad \text{3.5 meals per week could include indulgences}$$

If you are eating 3 meals per day (not quite up to eating every 3 hours yet, eh?) then it would be:

$$3 \quad \text{X} \quad 7 \quad = \quad \text{21 meals per week}$$

$$21 \quad \text{X} \quad 0.10 \quad = \quad \text{2.1 or 2 meals per week could include indulgences}$$

This is a great rule to remind us that no one should exclude the pleasures of food.

However, the only way that this rule can remain effective in getting you to your goals is if you keep it in perspective.

This is really important.

Eat without guilt AND jump right back on track after your indulgence.

Guilt is only useful if it catalyzes you to change at the next meal. Small doses of guilt can have a positive effect. However if you're beating yourself up because that's what you're practiced at doing and it isn't providing incentive to change, go back to week #3, *Stop Beating Yourself Up*.

You need to take action to change destructive behavior.

Jumping back on the wagon applies no matter what your breakdown of nutritious/indulgent food is. Even if you're averaging 50/50 throughout the holiday season, you still need to focus on getting back on track. If you don't, you're more likely to drop to 30/70 during the holidays.

90/10 calls for you to pay attention. By doing so, you can notice the point where the pleasure fades to 'I shouldn't be doing this.' Being able to recognize this shift in your mind is like illuminating a red signal, warning you that you need to stop the indulgence. The more practice that you get with mindful eating, which we talk about in week #11, the easier this will become. However, let's start you rolling with this: Make a commitment (in your mind or with your buddy) before you begin eating your delicacy of choice. Prime yourself by planning a personal experience in sensuality. Pay attention to the colors, textures, and flavour of what you're eating. Notice how it tastes at the different stages of chewing and as it moves through your mouth. While you're doing this, also tell yourself that you're going to notice at what point the pleasure shifts to guilt. When it does, you're going to stop.

'Oh yeah, sure,' you say? 'I'm going to stop eating black pepper and sea salt kettle chips before I consume half the bag?'

I promise that this gets easier with practice.

HOWEVER...

If you have certain foods that you find are near impossible to be moderate with, you have to make a decision. How much do you want to be at your ideal weight? What are you willing to do to have optimal health? What is the balance point for you between pleasure and your goals? It may be necessary to let these 'food vices' go completely, or to indulge in them only on the rare occasion. You have to weigh the consequences of your choice. Be honest with yourself. What happens when you indulge in that particular substance? (Don't be in denial if you are kettle chip addict and can't control yourself when they're in front of you). Decide if it's worth it and how many times you can handle the indulgence without losing your entire sense of control.

Those kettle chips I just mentioned, I love them. They're the only chips I crave and when I have them in my greasy little hands, I can't control myself. So here's what I've determined. Once every six months or so, I allow myself to bring a bag into the house and I know that until they are gone, I will be somewhat obsessive. After I eat them, I feel a bit unwell, not terrible, just not my usual. I have found a balance that works for me. The occasional pleasure is kept in perspective with the cost that it implies. More than a couple times a year will tip the balance too far off the level of health and self-control that I want for myself.

Another thing to pay attention to is how you feel after you indulge. If it makes you feel like crap, then remember the feeling. I mentioned this in the first week when I referred to motivation and your 'place of pain.' If you remember what it feels like to be in there, then you will want to indulge in the food that causes it, less and less. If you ignore your body and your pain, then you will have less powerful motivation to change.

Nourish Your Soul

What you need to do

The reality is, we often eat to soothe ourselves. If you just nodded your head, yes, that's true for me, then you need to find other 'sources of soothe.'

This is an important aspect of sustainable weight loss, because you need resources for feeling good that are at least as enticing as that initial high that you get from sugar, fats, breads, pasta, alcohol or your other favorite comfort food.

A part of this journey is about doing things that you love to do, that bring you joy, comfort and presence. Consider it a 'feeding of the soul'. Feeding the soul brings its own form of nourishment that we need to tap into on a daily basis. It balances us out, giving us a natural willpower that we don't have to work at.

The subject of 'feeding the soul' is particularly near and dear to my heart because it played a critical role in my own weight loss, and without me knowing it at the time, set me on a path to doing my life's work.

. . . .

When I was twenty-five, I was overweight and generally
dissatisfied with my life. I knew that I needed to shake
things up to get myself out of the stagnancy that had weaved

its way into my life. I booked myself for a six-month trip that included four and a half months in Africa. Being a Canadian girl who grew up in a middle class small town environment, it was transformative to experience a simpler way of living, one that is closer to the land, with its beauty and challenges, and in a continent that has political upheaval that is unlike anything that we know in Canada. It was eye opening and certainly shifted things around. However with all of newness that Africa offered me, the most life-changing experience was taking lots of images and falling in love with photography. I had not up to that point really explored my creativity. So after my travels, I moved from Vancouver to Victoria and embarked in a full-time program, immersing myself in both photography and as it happened, free dance. By day, I would spend my time shooting photos. At night, I was either in the darkroom or dancing freely in my spacious room. I was catalyzed into the excitement of getting up in the morning, of finally feeling fully alive. I pushed a lot of personal boundaries, took over ten thousand photos, danced nightly and journaled my thoughts. I ate smaller portions and never went for seconds because I was more excited about getting to my creative work. That was the year that I began the process of feeding my soul, freeing my mind, and sustainably losing the extra pounds.

Why you need to do it

You know the comfort that food provides, but you also know that the good feeling is not sustained. It dissipates rather quickly. Either you keep eating to make it last as long as you can or you drop into a more negative state than you were in before.

Behind the scenes, in a process that we are unconscious of while it's happening, the soothing is an attempt to get the good feeling that happens when the balanced brain chemistry of satisfaction, kicks into action.

I have mentioned these brain chemicals before, but it bears repeating now. Serotonin is the chemical that promotes a sense of wellbeing, dopamine gives us a boost of positive energy and generates a feeling of being rewarded, GABA calms us down, and the endorphins alleviate pain. In addition, oxytocin generates a sense of being loved and acetylcholine ensures that our cognitive abilities are on track. Deficiency of any of them can trigger cravings and overeating and an uncontrollable need to soothe the savage beast within.

The primary nutritional principles of this program are to eat protein and do it consistently throughout the day, mostly in companionship with vegetables, and to get enough good fat. Following those practices will go a long way to generating the raw materials needed to ensure an abundance of the happy neurochemicals. Exercise and rest play a part as well. But feeling good, soothing yourself, does not begin and end there.

By paying attention to the 'gap of awareness' you can find your own reasons for overeating. Whether it's stress, emotional discomfort or habitual triggers, you have a process of clarifying your personal brand of psychological hunger. When you can identify why you overeat, you can then decide what to do with that newfound awareness. Last week offered you ideas about emotional release. This week we need to talk about a different kind of nourishment that can relieve the ravages of stress and inner discomfort.

Feed your soul and you will enhance the production of those feel-good brain chemicals. You will also support the balance between the two hemispheres of the brain. The left side keeps you focused, prepared, and helps you maintain self-control. Too much time spent in this side of the brain however, leads to self-criticism, judgment, inflexibility, and an inability to see the larger picture. Feeding the soul taps you into the right side of the brain that is open, flexible, creative, compassionate, connected to the bigger picture. Also, if you are a believer and seeker of spiritual experiences, then this is the side of the brain that you want to spend some time in.

In a branch of psychology referred to as Positive Psychology, they have iden-tified the mental habits of those who more readily lose weight and keep it off and those who consistently struggle. If you are familiar with the way of thinking that goes like this; "I will be happy when I lose this weight," then you are tapping into a phenomenon that these psychologists have identified as the 'hedonic treadmill.' This is the human tendency to consistently seek something down the road or in the future, the "I'll be happy when..." way of thinking. The problem is that that kind of thinking leads to never being satisfied. Once you lose that weight, you still aren't happy because there is something else that you want. Maybe you want your hips to be thinner or your arms to be more toned or to look like your neighbour who is twenty years younger.

To beat your hedonic tendencies you need to focus on satisfaction in the moment. Finding what nourishes you now. Not tomorrow. Not yesterday. Not one year from now. Now.

In concept, this is simple. Find things that you love to do, that make you feel good, and you will have an easier route to heal your relationship with food and to lose weight in a way that seems easy and natural.

How you can do this

I was inspired by the idea of nourishing the soul a number of years ago when I read an article in a magazine. It asked its readership to share one of the activities that they do to lift their spirits. Out of all of the entries that were listed, the one that I recall was from a woman who wrote in to say that when she is stuck in traffic, she pulls a bubble container from the glove compartment, rolls down her window and blows bubbles at the other drivers. It makes them laugh, gives them ground for connection and lights up an otherwise boring drive. What struck me was the simplicity of her choice. For a few minutes in her day, at a time when she was stuck in a sit-uation not in her control, she chose to do something that lightens her own mood and spreads good will to those around her.

Sometimes we need to go out on a limb to feed our soul. We need to do something that pushes us outside of our comfort zone. For the woman above, she had to be willing to risk foolishness. But most of the time it only requires making a decision to prioritize this aspect of your wellbeing. In terms of the time commitment and the risk component, some soul-feeding activities will be easier for you. Go for the low hanging fruit, the stuff you can do easily and readily so that you can practice making it a daily occurrence. Then you can step into bigger projects, as you're ready.

Write down '30 things that feed your soul'.

Feeding your soul means that it brings you totally into the present moment, with no place else that you would rather be. If figuring out what nourishes you isn't obvious, as it isn't for many people, here are some ideas to consider:

Mindful and meditative activities – reading of spiritually inspiring books, prayer, listening to audios of guided meditation, chanting, three daily gratitudes, etc.

Pampering yourself – bubble baths, spa treatments, shopping, doing your own nails in beautiful colours, creating a new outfit with clothes in your closet, going to movies and/or concerts, etc.

Nature-based activities – lying on your back looking up at the clouds, going for walks on wooded trails, collecting shells, sitting or walking by the beach, watching the flow of a river, cross country skiing, hiking in the hills, making snow castles with your children, etc.

Creative endeavours – dancing to favourite songs, writing poems, blogging, listening to music, playing the piano, knitting, photo collaging, taking pictures, painting, etc.

Promotion of self-growth – attending lectures, reading inspiring books, philosophizing with friends, documentary films, journaling, taking a course just because you want to, etc.

Activities for fun and relaxation – hanging out with friends, exploring areas of the city you've never been, going on adventures with the children in your life, visiting art galleries, etc.

Generating love – playing with your cat, connecting with someone on a heart level, holding a baby, volunteer work, giving and getting a hug or a massage, talking with a close friend, doing something loving and unexpected for your mate, random acts of kindness, etc.

These are a few examples of the endless possibilities for feeding your soul. You need to consider what is personal and juicy for you. This will give you outlets that are more fulfilling and sustainable than comfort eating is.

If you can't find '30 things that feed your soul', don't fret. You're not alone. Remember that we get good at what we practice and if you are not practiced at self-nourishment, you have probably missed out on catching some of the opportunities to do so. As a result you're not even sure what works for you. Relax. Take some deep breaths. Seriously. Take some deep breaths right now.

It's okay to only have five or ten or even two. We all need to start from where we are and grow from there. Whatever number you have, you can take the next step.

Make a commitment to do at least one of the items on your list every single day.

Make your commitment doable so you have success at sticking with it. Maybe you will start with something that only takes three minutes like watching a funny video or listening to a song that moves you, or taking extra time to get down on the floor to play with your cat. With time, as you focus more and more on nourishing activities, the difference that you will feel in your well-being will be a motivating force to make it a daily practice.

Being in the practice of feeding your soul when you are not in the midst of a food craving, makes it easier to redesign your choices when you are facing emotional or habitual hunger. So don't wait to start. The time is now. Right now. Every time you give yourself the gift of feeding your soul, you are creating a brain pattern that is easier to return to, and will eventually replace food as your source of comfort and joy.

Week #9

. . . .

Rest and Relax to Lighten Up

. . .

Create a Healthy Relationship with Your Body

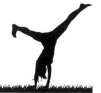

Rest and Relax to Lighten Up

What you need to do

Rest is a necessity for vital health. Yet, it is rarely mentioned in weight loss circles. This could be explained, at least in part, by the fact that the research connecting sleep and relaxation to being overweight is relatively new, and the maze of cause and effect is still to be determined. However there is a growing body of evidence pointing to an increase in weight in those who are sleep deprived and stressed out. To ignore rest means potentially blocking your chance of short or long term success. Experience has shown me the positive change that a conscious effort toward more restful states can have for some people – particularly (but not exclusively) for those who are stress eaters.

Once again, a reminder of one of the principles of *Jump Off the Diet Treadmill* – take it one step at a time. Small changes daily lead to big change over time. This whole-heartedly applies to getting more rest. Thirty minutes more of extra sleep or even a couple five minute rest periods during the day can have dramatic effect on your wellbeing and your relationship with food. So your focus for this week is to check in with your sleep patterns and your levels of energy during the day. If either needs enhancing, it is time to look for ways to do so.

Why you need to do this

In my professional practice in the financial district of Toronto, I have worked with a lot of highly ambitious people, male and female, who put rest at the bottom of their list of priorities. Many work sixty to seventy-five hours per week. They are often driven by high achievement and financial success. Although most also value their family, friends, health, fun, nature, and other outlets of fulfillment, they often get trapped in the spiral of heavy workloads and the expectations of their career. For them, and maybe for you, taking more time from your already busy schedule to relax during the day or to get more sleep, can seem like a pipe dream. The problem is however, adequate rest can be the determining factor for whether someone loses weight and keeps it off.

* *

I knew when I first shook Jane's hand that I was dealing with a powerhouse woman. Her handshake hinted at her strong, success-driven character. In addition to her seventy-hour workweek as an entrepreneurial consultant, she was also juggling single parenthood of three children after a painful divorce. She generally slept five hours and was going nonstop from morning to night.

Jane told me right off the hop that I should just tell her what to do and she would do it. She did prove to be compliant with her nutrition and exercise. She also demonstrated a willingness to address the issues behind her overeating. Still after three months she was frustrated that she had not lost much of the twenty pounds that she was desperate to shed. Her workload and her symptoms pointed in the direction of overtaxed adrenal glands, which meant an imbalance in cortisol levels that would ultimately cause her to stay heavy. I laid it out for her. Either slow down and 'smell the roses' or suffer the consequences of the stubborn belly fat that wasn't going anywhere and would likely expand with time. At that point, due to an excessive workload and her children's full schedule, she nodded her understanding and then proceeded to do nothing about finding a better work/rest balance.

In subsequent sessions I continued to harp the importance of 'chilling out' and sleeping more. Finally, with the pain of not successfully losing weight deepening her motivation, she made a point of clearing her summer schedule so that she could take two months off to spend time with the kids at their cottage and to take care of herself. She hired a yoga teacher to create a routine for her, I reminded her of how to do BLMS and gave her a series of journaling exercises. At the end of the summer, she came back to the coaching. She had lost six pounds despite the extra indulgences in wine and berry pies (she had loved to bake with her Mom as a kid – the summer had also been a time to reinstill her love of pie-making.) She looked lighter – both physically and energetically. Her face was radiant. The challenge now was to incorporate restful activities into her schedule once she was back at work and the kids were back in school and extracurricular activities.

Although she had moments that she fell off the 'rest wagon', she had experienced the difference that taking time out and more sleep had made not only to her waistline but also to her sense of wellbeing. She scheduled in yoga classes twice a week and promised to take two fifteen-minute breaks everyday just to breath, meditate or listen to music. In essence to practice doing 'nothing'. She also committed to being in bed by eleven o'clock, five out of seven nights. It wasn't always easy but she was getting better at each of these practices. After two years of ups and downs, but consistent effort to change her work schedule (she now keeps it to fifty hours per week) and to practice her 'nothingness' as she affectionately called it, she has shed fifteen of those twenty pounds and is happy that she is moving in the right direction.

Unfortunately some people never get their head around the benefits that would be gleaned by taking more time in each day to be restful. They haven't made a strong enough connection, intellectually and/or experientially between the lack of sleep and relaxation, and their weight.

It makes sense that we would gain weight under consistent sleep deprivation if we look at our primitive hardwiring. Our prehistoric genes see sleep deprivation as a response to a threat. (Why else would we ever deprive ourselves of sleep or relaxation time?) Threat equals stress. What happens under stress? We store body fat to ensure that we have enough fuel to survive, while we are running and fending off our attacker. (Remember this is primitive.) That may not be a problem if it happens occasionally, for short periods of time. But combine years of sleep deprivation with modern workloads and you have a lifestyle ripe for consistent weight gain.

What is considered 'sleep deprivation?' Before Thomas Edison gifted us with added light we would sleep ten to fourteen hours per night, as our circadian clock was adjusted to the lack of daytime light. In modern times, research varies on what constitutes adequate sleep. There is room for individual needs – creative people and those who nap during the day may need less. For the average person, anywhere between six and a half to nine hours has been identified as enough sleep. However the research linking sleep deprivation to weight gain or its potential in young adults is generally noted at five hours or less. There is also a detrimental effect at six hours, albeit it seems to be proportionally less.

The Nurses Health Study followed more than 68,000 women over a six-teen-year period having them self-report on their hours of sleep. While adjusting for other factors such as exercise and diet, it was discovered that those who slept five hours or less per night were fifteen percent more likely to become obese in those years than those who slept seven hours or more. Those who slept six hours were at a six percent greater risk of obesity.

A Wisconsin sleep study of 1,024 people made the association between short sleep duration and an alteration in the appetite regulating hormones, leptin and ghrelin. Leptin is the hormone that elevates our sense of sati-ation and metabolism. For participants who slept five hours, their leptin levels were 15.5 percent lower. The levels of ghrelin, the hormone that fuels our appetite, making us seek food, was 14.9 percent higher in the five-hour sleepers vs. the eight-hour sleepers.

Our twenty-four hour circadian rhythms that determine our day and nighttime cycles are regulated by the suprachiasmatic nucleus (SCN), a big name for a little rice-sized organ in the hypothalamus of the brain. The SCN is in communication with other parts of the brain and various other organs such as the liver, heart, intestines, the retina of the eye as well as fat cells. All of these parts work together to modulate sleep, body temperature, as well as the release of hormones. Beyond that, the SCN, our circadian clock, influences nearly all aspects of physiology and behaviour. If we alter the rhythmic pattern that is generated by the SNC and its 'slave' tissues, then we may be potentially playing with metabolic fire. The wirings of the human body are intricate, complex and beyond my full comprehension or the parameters of this book. However to support the 'why' of sleep, let's look at some of the hormones that are woven into the workings of the SCN and our sleep, rest, and weight patterns.

Leptin and Ghrelin – I already mentioned these hormones that influence satiation and appetite, respectively. We need adequate amounts of leptin to be in a state of food calm, to not feel the constant pull of hunger. And ghrelin is there to ensure that we don't starve ourselves. It kicks in to up our appetite. Alterations in sleep patterns are being associated with de-creases in leptin and increases in ghrelin. The result? You guessed it. We want to eat more.

Insulin and Glucose – You may recall from week #6, *Check Those Simple Carbs at the Door* that glucose is the simplest form of sugar that the body and brain use for fuel and insulin is the hormone that helps to shuttle glucose from the bloodstream into the cells. Eve Van Cauter, PhD, a scientist at the University of Chicago, and her team found that deep sleep deprivation could alter insulin levels and glucose metabolism quite dramatically. In one study, nine healthy young adults between the ages of 20 and 31, who slept under clinical observation for five nights, were, for three of those nights, disturbed by sounds whenever they entered the restorative deep sleep cycle. The disturbance to these periods of sleep mimicked the changes that often happen as we age. In essence, their sleep became equivalent to that of a 60 year old. The results are quoted from the press release regarding the study: "...after only three nights of selective slow-wave sleep suppression, young healthy subjects became less sensitive to insulin. Although they needed more insulin to dispose of the same amount of glucose, their insulin secretion did not increase to compensate for the reduced sensitivity, resulting in reduced tolerance to glucose and increased risk for type 2 diabetes. The decrease in insulin sensitivity was comparable to that caused by gaining 20 to 30 pounds." Van Cauter has stated that sleep deprivation is the 'royal route to obesity' due to its long term effects on health and weight.

Cortisol – This hormone influences your state of arousal, and so in a healthy person, is at its peak when you wake up and slows down production as the day wears on. At bedtime it should be at its lowest levels. Cortisol is involved in blood sugar regulation, the stress response and in keeping fat stored in your fat cells. Too much cortisol equals too much fat, especially around the abdomen. If you do not find time to relax during the day, your body may stay in a continuous state of arousal (stress response), leading to fluctuating cortisol levels throughout the day, possibly ending the day with high levels. People who have trouble with insomnia are more likely to have abnormal cortisol levels which peak in the hours before bed and the wee hours of the night rather than in the morning. Balancing out-of-whack cortisol levels demands more relaxation time during the day as well as appropriate sleep hygiene.

Melatonin – Melatonin is intricately tied into our circadian rhythm of day and night. It increases in the hours of darkness, in preparation for our bedtime. Melatonin enhances the immune system, provides support as an anti-cancer agent, and acts as an antioxidant to protect the fatty tissue of the brain. In relation to our weight loss journey, it is needed to lower cortisol levels while we sleep, which means more opportunity for fat cell normalization.

Human Growth Hormone – HGH is our restorative hormone for the muscle, organs, bone, and immune tissues. In fact it affects almost every cell in the body and is considered the ultimate anti-aging hormone. In relation to fat loss, it supports the building of muscle, which acts like a furnace in our body, burning more calories at rest than fatty tissue. HGH also frees up stored body fat to use it as a source of fuel. Unfortunately HGH production gets less and less with age, decreasing by fourteen percent per decade, so by the time we reach our sixties we are operating on eighty percent less HGH. This has been implicated in the aging and decline of our bodies. Optimal HGH production depends on deep sleep between the hours of 11 pm to 2 am, as well as stabilizing blood sugar levels throughout the day and getting regular moderately strenuous exercise.

Serotonin – Deep sleep restores our levels of serotonin, the feel good neurotransmitter that regulates appetite, mood, assertiveness, pain, sexual behaviour, and sleep. It also is a major force behind our cravings for sweets and fats. Too much stress (and cortisol levels that are too high) leads to the amino acid tryptophan, which produces serotonin, being used for other purposes. This causes serotonin levels to fall. Thus the importance of getting deep sleep and committing to time for relaxation throughout an otherwise busy day.

Research also connects sleep deprivation to impairment of activity in the prefrontal cortex of the brain. This is the area where decision making and willpower happen. It seems that too little sleep over time will alter our food selections towards foods that are high in sugar and fat as opposed to those that are healthy, such as vegetables.

In addition to the circadian clock and its affect on the twenty-four hour cycle, our brains and bodies also establish ultradian rhythms. These are patterns that occur more frequently throughout the day. There are many different ultradian rhythms. As an example both heart rate and temperature are regulated in cyclical patterns. But I want to draw your attention to one particular rhythm. It is the ninety to 120 minute cycle of left brain/

right brain activity. The cycle goes something like this: for ninety minutes most of us are operating primarily in the left side of the brain, which is logical, analytical, and detail oriented. It allows us to focus on language, numbers, research and routine tasks, what might be called 'at your desk' type of work. After those ninety minutes, there is approximately twenty minutes in which a shift happens to the right side of the brain. From here we can experience daydreaming, creativity, intuition, and a big-picture focus. If we ignore our need to break from more routine activities to be receptive to uncontrolled, creative thinking, or to rest and relax, we can deplete our energy and productivity. It can also affect the balance of the feel-good hormones such as dopamine, serotonin and GABA that generate our level of happiness. Imagine a day in which you have no rest from the routine, no point in the day that you take those breaks. (Most of us can relate to many, many days like that). At those times, are you more likely to turn to food to boost your energy and your sense of pleasure? Oh yeah – here comes that mid-afternoon latte and cookie.

How you can do it

Consider the infamous 'to-do list'. Whether yours is in written form or clearly located in one of the recesses of your mind, it is limitless. It is like a creature that continues to grow, constantly having to be fed more and more tasks. These are tasks that the creature isn't going to do. You are. And it's not like you are going to do a task and you never have to do it again. I have always been amazed at how I can clean the kitchen floor, and within three days, it needs cleaning again.

Think of it – when was the last time that you can remember, when you sat down and said to yourself – "oh good, there's nothing that I need to do. I can take a break now and rest until something else shows up". HA! If you wait for the moment when there is nothing to do, you will never rest.

You have to prioritize relaxation time. Time that is devoted, unadulterated and committed to relaxation. No phone calls, children, spouses, or office duties to interrupt. It might only need to be a few three-minute periods of deep breathing, or a thirty-minute walk in the park, or a twenty-minute nap. However if you can give it more time, do. The space in your mind expands with the increase in time given.

My suggestion is, as it is with all of the other components of this program, start with one step at a time. Make it doable. Avoid making your relaxation period into another task on your 'to do' list that you may or may not get to. Start with what you can handle. Consult the 'Relaxation Propositions' below for ideas of short and longer options for relaxation.

Here is what happens when you do. First, you will quickly shift yourself into the relaxation side of your autonomic (automated) nervous system. The difference will be palpable. You will feel calmer, softer, and will be able to return to your tasks with more focus. Second, you will be honoring yourself and your body by doing something purely for the sake of your health. Every time you do something that's good for you, you strengthen your self-esteem and self-respect. You make a statement that you and your body matter – enough so that you will take a break or a few breaks in the day to give your body what it needs.

Likewise your choice to be in bed by 10:00 or 10:30 in order to ensure a good night's sleep is supporting the same commitment to yourself and your body. It says, 'my health is my priority. Only with good health will I function at my peak and be able to accomplish more than I could possibly do now.'

Sleep Factors

The circadian clock is synchronized with changes in environment, temperature, light, and rituals. Let's categorize some of the factors that will influence optimal snooze time. You can check to see which ones might be affecting your own state of restfulness. If you want to track your patterns, you can download a 'sleep journal' from the resources page of my website at www.foodcoach.ca.

Retiring Time – Entrain your sleep clock by going to bed at the same time each night. That way your body will be expecting it. The period of 10:00 pm to 2:00 am is the time that is the most rejuvenating as the levels of melatonin rise to their peak at around midnight. It is also when our sleep is the deepest. Ideally develop a routine of retiring as close to 10:00 pm as you can. You can do this by committing yourself to retiring earlier in fifteen-minute increments.

Having said that, some people are confirmed night owls and will probably not ever reach a 10:00 pm retirement. Nor should they, necessarily. There is research to show that people who are more productive in the evening hours and go to bed later have more flexibility in their circadian clock. They seem to have more internal control and depend less on the rise and fall of light to determine their sleep/wake cycle. Whether you are early-to-bed, early-to-rise or a late-night person, the other factors of good sleep need to be considered to ensure steady sleep for a minimum of 6.5 hours. And if you continue to struggle with your weight despite good efforts in every other area, you may want to consider rearranging your priorities to get to bed earlier.

Food eaten during the day and within 3 hours of retiring – Given the dance of hormones that goes on at night to activate your sleep patterns, ensuring that you are stabilizing and fueling those chemicals is imperative to good sleep. There are no hard fast rules around eating before bed. My experience is that some people do better going to sleep having not eaten three hours prior. Other people need food within thirty to sixty minutes prior to sleep to help stabilize their blood sugar through the night. Often those folks will also need to eat consistently throughout the day, every three hours or so, including lots of protein, vegetables and good fat to support the normalized function of insulin, glucose and the other fuel regulating hormones.

* *

John is a client who, like many, came to me to lose weight. When I asked him about his sleep, he shared that he had struggled with it for as long as he could remember. He often woke up at around 3 am and couldn't get back to sleep for a couple of hours. He would think over whatever legal case he was working on. He might get back to sleep at around 5 am, one hour before he had to get up for the day. This had been going on for years. The sleep clinic hadn't been able to help his situation. A review of his diet showed that he was erratic in his eating, obsessively focused on low calories and he finished eating at around 6:30 pm but typically didn't go to bed until midnight. I discussed the importance of stabilizing his hormones and set him up to make change to do so, including having a nighttime snack that was rich in protein, fat and fibre. Within one week of consistent eating, he reported that he was sleeping through the night, averaging six hours. Even better, a couple weeks later, he had committed to retiring one or even two hours earlier, and was thrilled to be getting closer to seven or eight hours of uninterrupted sleep. He also shed fifteen pounds over a three month period. That was impressive for a guy who hadn't slept well for at least twenty years.

Here are some food options before bed that could help to stabilize your blood sugar:

- Cottage cheese or ricotta cheese sprinkled with hemp or chia seeds
- Dense whole grain (rye, spelt, kamut, gluten free) bread with organic peanut butter or almond butter
- Chia Wonder Cereal (recipe on www.foodcoach.ca) or a nut and seed based granola (keep it to a maximum of five grams of sugar per serving) or a muesli with Greek yogurt or a protein shake (recipes on my website)
- Natural Factors makes a meal replacement called SlimStyles that has PGX fibre in it. Have one of those as a shake or make it into a pudding by blending it with milk and placing it in the fridge for at least one hour. Read more about PGX in week #12, *Consider Researched Supplements.*
- Any of the snacks listed in week #2, *Eat Breakfast and Keep Eating* that appeal to you will do.

Activities within one hour before bed – Working on the computer or watching TV emits too much light for optimal melatonin levels to be secreted. Also, the body responds to clear signals that bedtime is approaching, thus the importance of rituals that separate the activity of the day from night-time sleep. This is where an evening walk, a bath, reading fiction or some pre-bed stretching can be the clue to relax your body and mind and ready it for sleep. On the other hand, falling asleep in front of the TV lacks the clarity of 'daytime ends and sleep time begins'.

Bedroom Environment – Ensure that your bedroom is sufficiently darkened to support a strong output of melatonin. Electromagnetic fields as well as the light emanating from electronic devices can affect a sensitive person, even if you're not conscious of the affect. Inadequate window coverings may allow too much ambient light to seep into the room. If you have tried everything else and could still use some improvement to your sleep, this would be worth addressing to see if it helps. Also, if you are sensitive to sounds and/or to the chaos of a disorganized bedroom, both need to be addressed if you are going to snooze effectively.

Emotional/mental load – People who are emotionally sensitive seem to suffer more from sleep deprivation due to worry and obsessing over their thoughts and feelings. Deep dream states are times that we work through some of our emotional issues and emotionally sensitive people may not be using that dreamtime to their advantage if their sleep is disrupted. There is an increase in the depletion of the feel-good hormone serotonin, which is reliant on deep sleep for its restoration. This translates into a greater susceptibility to poor decision making around food and more emotional eating to try to boost serotonin and counter the stress. It is imperative to have outlets for emotional release that give you relief from worry and obsessive thinking. Go to week # 7, *Take Charge of Your Emotions* for more support in this area.

For those who have a lot on your mind that keeps you awake ruminating, you'll need to develop some strategies to help with this. Make a list of 'to do's' for the next day so you're not thinking about it during the wee hours. Other forms of writing to get clarity and focus can be powerful. Creating a clear boundary between day and nighttime activities, as mentioned before, is a crucial practice. Meditation during the day or quiet activities before bed can be helpful. The one thing that is best avoided right before bed is work or the subject that you are thinking most about. You need to make a clear demarcation line before bed.

'Relaxation Propositions'

I am challenging you to learn to relax by using one or more of the techniques listed below. These ideas are intended to change your physiology and behavior in a substantial way by learning to do less, or maybe nothing at all. Choose something that you know is doable and for the next three weeks practice it everyday (or at least, most days) so that you reinforce it and can turn it into a habit.

Give yourself a pat on the back, an acknowledgment, for engaging in any of the relaxation techniques below. Note how you feel when you do it, and afterwards.

Deep breathing – 1 to 3 minutes. Imagine that you have a hollow bamboo tube running from the top of your head to the base of your spine. As you inhale through your nose, draw the breath all the way to the bottom of the tube and then back up again and then out on your exhale. Do this at least ten times. There are many other ways to breath consciously. Choose this one or another that you know of. Deep breathing is the quickest way to shift us into the relaxation side of our autonomic nervous system.

Eye rest – 2 to 3 minutes. Cover your eyes with your hands, an eye pillow or with slices of cucumber (oh, so cooling!). Deep breathe while you're doing it. This is particularly good if you suffer from eyestrain caused by staring at a screen all day, or you have allergies that cause irritation to the eyes. But you can also do it just because it feels good to do so.

Quiet time – 5 to 60 minutes. Reading, contemplating, being out in nature, looking up at the clouds, doing nothing. TV doesn't count because it fills your mindspace with noise and directs your thinking, rather than providing freedom for you to create space in your mind.

Napping – 20 or 90 minutes. I have a favourite napping technique that takes twenty minutes and always gives me a second wind. Lay on the floor, with your lower legs supported by a chair so they are at a ninety-degree angle. Put a rolled up towel under your neck and lower back so all of your weight is supported. Cover yourself with a blanket if you might get chilled. Put headphones on with relaxing music and set an alarm for twenty minutes. See if this isn't the most productive short rest period that you've ever had. Note that a nap shouldn't exceed thirty minutes unless you can occasionally do a long one at ninety minutes. Between thirty and ninety minutes, you get into brain wave patterns that will make you feel drowsy when you awaken from them.

Meditation – 10 to 60 minutes. There are many forms of meditation and any of them would be fine. If you need to learn how to do it, you can browse, 'how to meditate' online and choose one or more techniques that speak to you. One of the easiest forms is mediation 'music' that taps into what are called binaural beats. These sound tracks shift us into the trance-like, calming brain wave patterns that increase relaxation, creativity, focus, and spirituality. It helps alter our brainwave patterns quicker than regular meditation. I particularly like Kelly Howell's meditations (www.brainsync.com) or Omharmonics downloads and community orientation (www. omharmonics.com).

Walking with intention – 5 to 60 minutes. This can include different forms of moving meditation, such as deep breathing, listening to music or observational walking (as in noticing beautiful gardens, rocks, buildings, etc).

Music concentration – 3 minutes or more. With headphones on, focus on the specific sounds within the 'musicscape'. Choose an instrument to follow, dissect the lyrics or the arrangements. This is its own form of meditation but it can also be combined with walking and the napping technique mentioned above. Or let the music move you into free dance.

Spending time in nature – 3 minutes or more. Research has shown that nature calms down the prefrontal cortex of our brain where our decision-making and willpower happen. In essence, nature creates more 'space' in your mind so that you can have greater control over your choices. The more time the better, but even staring at a tree outside your window can have a beneficial effect.

Yoga, Tai Chi, Aikido or another contemplative form of movement – 10 to 90 minutes. There is a difference between standard forms of exercising where you are working assertively to build muscle or increase your cardiovascular heath, and mindful forms of movement that help you slow down your mind while you exercise your body. The goals are different but equally important. If you have trouble being still for the sake of relaxation, contemplative movement is a great option.

A final note:

Hormone fluctuations that are happening during the day and night will have an effect on your nighttime patterns. If you are addressing all of the factors mentioned above and still struggle with your energy levels and sleep cycles, then it would be worth having your physiology checked by a professional who deals with functional medicine. I make further references to this in my addendum on *10 Physical Issues that will Stop You from Losing Weight (Despite Your Best Efforts).*

Create a Healthy Relationship
With Your Body

What you need to do

I have discovered that many people cannot connect to their body from the neck down. Their awareness is focused only in their head. Yet the body is constantly channeling information to us, if we choose to pay attention. By listening, your body will guide you to your ideal diet and lifestyle, allowing for alterations and adaptations as your needs demand. On the other hand, ignore your body and it will go into innumerable forms of pain trying to get your attention.

This week is about beginning (or deepening) your practice of listening to your body. From listening, you will develop trust, and from trust, respect. That is the foundation of any healthy relationship.

Why you need to this

Without access to your body's messages, you miss out on some important information that will clarify your thoughts, feelings, dreams and intuitions. As well, the wisdom of your body will relay info about what, when, why and how you need to eat. With practice, you can find a personal diet that is ideal for you at any given time, rather than being vulnerable to the whims of media, the weight loss industry and food marketers. You can also take it beyond diet to recognize other factors that enhance or drain your energy, are the cause of symptoms, and those that alter your mood.

Not liking your body is a heavy burden to carry. Think of it as energetic weight. Metaphorically, it is similar to any relationship. If there is someone in your family, your circle of friends or a work colleague with whom you share an unresolved dislike (or even if it's one-sided), the air will be thick with tension when you are together. Now consider the fact that you are always with your body. It has been with you from the moment of birth and together you go, to your last breath. That is long time to carry the weight of inharmonious tension. No wonder people disconnect from the neck down. They don't want to be reminded of the dysfunctional relationship that they have with their constant companion.

As you have been reading through the ideas and practices in this book, I hope it has become clear that *Jump Off the Diet Treadmill* involves an understanding of you as a whole connected being, not just a mind isolated from your body. Losing weight needs to happen not only physically, but also emotionally, mentally and spiritually. To live in a balanced, healthy, and light body, we need to connect those pieces of the puzzle. But to do that, we first need to break down the parts to make it accessible and do-able. The body gives us a way in to all of those parts. As grounded as it is, it offers us direct access to our emotions and a way to release them. If we 'get into' the body and give it what it needs, it helps us clarify our needs and wants. And from my perspective, one that you can choose to pursue or not, it offers the most profound inroads into spirituality. It is somewhat ironic that by being grounded in the physical, in the present moment, connected to the senses, that we have greater access to life beyond the containment of our body.

Without body awareness – health, peace of mind, playfulness, happiness, and wisdom are less accessible. This is because the mind alone cannot be trusted. It tells stories and believes those stories to be true. Yet that truth is often based on experiences from the past and desires for the future but not the reality of the present. But the body, with its primal language of the senses informs the mind and provides invaluable information that keeps us grounded in the moment. It is from this place that we can now choose how to respond to what is before us. The past can't be changed (other than our perspective on it), nor the future (other than in our minds where we plan and dream). It is the ever-present moment from which we can take responsibility to change what doesn't serve us or accept what can't be changed. The best way (I believe it to be the only way) to be in the moment is to be connected to the language of the body.

Most people who have struggled with their weight want a positive body image, as well as a sense of freedom within their body. If you have a strong self-esteem but a poor body image, you want the outside appearance to be in sync with how you feel inside. You want your body to be a reflection of your character. If however, you still lack confidence in your character, there is work to be done to gain that confidence, and then to match the inside with the outside. In both cases, the communication with your body is crucial.

How you can do it

The brain works by creating a series of body maps that are networks of neural pathways woven together throughout the brain and body. Amongst other things we have body maps for our 'body schema', which is our experience of our body in space. As an example, knowing how much of the doorway we will need as we walk through it, how big or small we are next to another person, how much weight we generate when we sit in a chair are experiences of the body schema. We are of course, unconscious of this body map as we are of all of them, but they are there. Another series of maps that we have created are the ones that form our 'body image'. Rather than being about our body in physical space as is the body schema maps, body image is our *perception* of how our body looks. We strengthen our body image maps when we look in the mirror and make judgments, good or bad, about our appearance.

When you lose weight you will likely experience a change in your body schema – you feel greater ease as your body goes up the stairs, the tops of your thighs don't rub together, you take up less room in a crowded subway. However for some people, their body image doesn't change. So even though you now weigh less, you might still see yourself as the fat person in the heavier body. The problem is of course, that the two maps need to eventually create harmonious connections or you will remain in a state of internal conflict. If you continue to perceive yourself as a fat person, despite being thinner, the conflict in your brain will resolve itself in one of two ways: either you will become physically fat again, or your body image transforms to reflect the change in your physical appearance. Then you will match your internal image with your external schema. A couple of examples might help to clarify the difference.

A number of years back, I worked with Darla, a lovely woman in her early fifties. She had struggled in her relationship with food and her body for as long as she could remember. It was clear from our conversations that she carried a great deal of 'baggage' from her past, particularly from her relationship with her mother. Her mom passed on a consistent message – that Darla was fat. She had her go on diets starting when she was five. She was sent to the family doctor many times with the conversation always turning to weight loss. She was even shipped off to fat camp when she was eleven. The irony is, that when she looks back at photos of herself as a child and teen, Darla can see that she was a bit plump, but certainly not fat. In the first six months of our work together, she was eating consistently throughout the day, diminished her dependency on sweets, lost fifteen pounds and was 'singing my praises,' but not her own. Slowly but surely, her resolve to take care of herself diminished. She would get too busy to eat, couldn't prioritize walking or going to yoga. Despite my encouragement and unconditional support, she berated herself for being weak and lazy. She actually was neither. She worked hard. She had the accomplishments of a master's degree, an art collection, a successful business. Weak and lazy she was not. But she would not make the commitment to giving herself the time and focus to learn to listen to her body, to trust what it was saying to her and to respect it enough to take the time to create change. Her inner landscape remained the same and thus so did the perspectives that kept her heavy.

On the opposite side of the fence, you may recall Susan, the executive coach in her forties who had been sexually abused as a child. I introduced her in week #7, Take Charge of Your Emotions. Here is a woman whose body had been a huge source of pain for her. But she recognized that in order to reach her goals, to heal, to become free, she needed to connect with her body, to learn to love it. As mentioned, she had done a lot of therapy by the time she had come to work with me, so she was ready for one more link in the chain of healing. Now she was looking for something that challenged her to take on her physicality rather than to run away from it. She was persistent in the work that she did – free dancing, writing, yoga, walks in nature. Whatever she needed, she would make the time to prioritize it. What evolved was a total shift in her relationship with her body, so that even with the extra weight that she carried, she was seeing herself as a lighter person. Her body image shifted before her physical weight, but it eventually followed.

The idea of 'body image' is based on your perceptions. Your perceptions are based on past experiences, parental, societal and media influences, and the beliefs about your body that you have formed from that history. Changing your body image requires a shift in perspective.

Let's start with where you are at right now.

Describe your relationship with your body, in one to three lines:

If you have trouble imagining your relationship with your body, try this visualization:

Get comfortable. Close your eyes. Take ten deep breaths, focusing on the movement of the breath in and out of your body.

Now imagine that you are in a room. This room is designed to your liking, with the colors, temperature, furniture and surroundings that you choose.

In this room are two comfy chairs side by side. You sit down in one chair and in the other you invite the entity of your body to sit.

Notice what form your body shows up as. Trust how it shows up. There is no right or wrong. Your imagination can inform you.

How does your body look? (Big, small, wiry, see-through, blubbery, wrapped up, chained...?)

What energy does it exude? (Happiness, shame, joy, anger, fear, embarrassment...?)

What does your body want to tell you? Ask it to speak to you and tell you what it feels.

Then ask your body what you can do for it right now, in this moment?

Finally, ask you body if there is anything else that it wants to say to you?

When you are finished your visualization, write down your experience.

What makes any relationship one that is healthy and loving?

I would wager a guess that most of us would agree that these provide a foundation:

- Trust
- Respect
- Open and honest communication

Would you say that how you described your body, reflects love, trust and respect?

Trust and respect develop from open communication.

Let's look at how we can develop that open communication with our body.

It happens in two ways: by listening to what it has to say, and by speaking to it in a loving and respectful way.

Listening to your body

The raw materials of the body's language are the senses: hearing, sight, touch, taste and smell.

Metaphorically, they are the words of body language. The stories that the body weaves are relayed to us via our energy, mood and symptoms. When you have an abundance of vitality, contentment, and a body that is free of pain or sickness, then you know you are treating your containment vehicle well. On the other hand, a lack of zest, joy and mobility are messages to pay attention. Let's take a closer look at the stories the body tells:

Energy

If you are listening to your body and giving it what it needs, one of the ways it rewards you, is through energy. The ideal of course, is to have your energy steady and consistently high throughout the day and into the evening, within an hour or two of retiring for the night. If your energy is lagging, your body is giving you a clear message that there is something you need to pay attention to.

Energy can be generated or drained in numerous ways: physically, emotionally, mentally or spiritually.

Physically, are you eating the foods that provide the needed raw materials for your body and brain: protein, good fats, vitamins, minerals, enzymes, and water? Are you fueling it with the complex carbohydrates? Or, on the other hand, are you feeding it manufactured foods that have hidden chemicals and toxic substances? These processed foodstuffs can mimic and replace real nutrients in the structure of the cells and tissues. They will then alter your metabolism. If nutrition is an issue for you, go back through weeks one to seven of this program, one step at a time, to be reminded about how you can change your dietary lifestyle.

Another way that you will physically drain your energy is by not resting enough. Both sleep deprivation and a lack of relaxation throughout the day will alter hormone and electrical signals that influence metabolism. If you struggle with rest, be sure to read and take action on the info in this week's notes on rest and relaxation.

Finally, regarding physical energy, you will do yourself no service to ignore your body's need for movement. Exercise powerfully propels metabolism, charging the cells to produce energy. You can't help but notice the change almost immediately, especially if you go from sitting on your butt in front of the computer to some form of movement.

> *In writing this book, I have been staring at the screen for hours in a day, and have been doing it for months. At the moment that I'm writing this, I'm slouching like an aged sloth. Signal computes. Need movement. Switch to iTunes. Choose music that I'm in the mood for. Black Keys? The Heavy? Marvin Gaye? Dance like a banshee for three songs. Supercharge!! Back to writing with a renewed perspective, better posture and way more energy than I had ten minutes before.*

If exercise is a problem for you, week #4, *Find the Exercise that is Right for You* will provide some support.

In relation to the emotions, having hidden closets in your mind in the form of secrets and dark recesses, takes a lot of energy to maintain. Those closets are filled with all forms of illusions, perceptions and beliefs. They are the cellular storage places of memories that are unconsciously driving your thoughts and behaviors. If you think that you can keep those doors closed for good and still have great energy, think again. Your body is telling you to clear the space to make room for clarity and focus, which are energy generating, rather than draining. If emotions are something that you need help releasing, turn to week #7, *Take Charge of Your Emotions*.

Your body feels the mental energy drain when your mind is not being stimulated through learning and creativity. Also when you choose to *not* give your analytical, logical, detail and task oriented side of the brain periodic breaks in the day, down goes your energy, like a drain sucking the fluids from your brain cavity. Look to week #3, *Stop Beating Yourself Up*, week #8, *Nourish Your Soul* and this week re: rest and relaxation, for more support on strengthening your mental energy.

Spiritually, you will lose energy if you are not on purpose in fulfilling your life. Ultimately *Jump Off the Diet Treadmill* is about greater freedom, awareness, and self-development. By bringing you into a deeper relationship with your body and yourself, you are creating a foundation for a purposeful life. Follow your soul to engage in activities that keep you passionate and present in the moment. Go to week #8, *Nourish the Soul*. As an added resource, on my website under resources, I have posted an adaptation of some writing by Marc David, the founder of the Institute for the Psychology of Eating (www.psychologyofeating.com) called Core Life Lessons. This speaks more directly to the challenges of spirit that you may need to address.

Mood

Parallel to energy levels, the body communicates its needs through mood. All areas that affect energy also challenge your disposition.

Physically, mood will be a reflection of the neurotransmitters and hormones that are directly related to reward, pleasure, satisfaction and happiness. Dopamine, serotonin, endorphins, GABA and acetylcholine all need the right raw materials to function properly. Also a consistent supply of fuel to the brain in the form of complex carbs and protein to stabilize your blood sugar is imperative to a steady nature. Thus once again, nutrition sets the stage for how your body will communicate with you.

Emotional stability will be reflected by a steadiness of character and positive outlooks. Unattended baggage can cause explosions of temper. In times of negativity, emotional drama, and underlying sadness, the body is relaying the need to pay attention. This was explained more thoroughly in week #7, *Take Charge of Your Emotions*.

Excitement and enthusiasm naturally accompanies a cheery mood. The lack of something that stimulates you mentally and/or spiritually can lead to depression or some variance of it. Follow the paths mentioned previously under energy to discover ways to alter your moods by way of soulfulness, rest and creativity.

Symptoms

Any form of symptom can be a message that your body needs something it's not getting, or less of something that it's getting too much of. As an example, if you are overweight, you may have accompanying inflammation in the body that can show up as pain in the joints, problems with digestion, headaches, difficulty breathing, or any number of other symptoms. Ignoring these messages will deepen the problems and lead to you living with constant pain. Your norm is one far below the line of optimal health. An exploration of what might be triggering symptoms should include an assessment of food intolerances, and with the help of a professional, a review of other possible imbalances that might be causing the problem.

Andrea came to me not only needing to lose weight but to deal with the crazy mental fog, moodiness and anxiety that had been getting worse with time. She had shortness of breath, low energy, intense sugar and carb cravings, night sweats, constant aches, and an unquenchable thirst. Andrea suspected that she had a wheat allergy but the doctors and dietician that she went to said that it wasn't likely to be a concern. They thought it was 'all in her head' and said so. So for years she has been ignoring the messages from her body despite her intuition.

In the first few weeks that we started working together I supported her to follow her instinct (I think Andrea would attest that I did so emphatically), explaining how her food intolerances could be causing a lot of her symptoms. She was motivated to eliminate all of the wheat from her diet, replacing it with other whole grains and beans. I also suggested that she eat every three hours, including some protein, to maintain hormonal balance.

The client review that she sent me the following week included this, and I quote "I don't feel depressed. I don't feel life is hopeless! I feel a new sense of joy and hope! I truly can't get over the change in how I feel! I have energy to do things. I don't want to sit around because I feel so ill. It is a reality – food has a HUGE impact on the mental, physical and spiritual aspects of myself."

Wow. I couldn't have said it better.

Andrea's experience is common. With attention to points of dysfunction and a willingness to address them, transformation can happen fast. I have seen it many times, where a change in diet along with perspective shifts can alter a person's digestive tract, improve their sleep and up their energy within a few weeks. However, ignore the signals long enough and you can potentially cause irreversible damage. At that point only dramatic intervention in the form of surgery or lifetime use of pharmaceutical drugs will provide any relief.

There are also layers to address when paying attention to symptoms. The first layer is the physical. Get yourself out of pain first so you can focus on more detailed messages from the body. While you are addressing the direct influences on symptoms via nutrition, rest and movement, you can also tune into the mental and emotional layers to explore what is being communicated there. Finally, address your spirit.

A lovely older woman approached me at the end of a seminar I gave on sustainable weight loss. She wanted to know if I could help her if she came to see me in the clinic. She had been trying to lose weight that was centered in her belly and had been to a number of practitioners including a well-known local naturopath. They had done extensive lab tests, had given her lots of supplements, corrected her diet but ultimately there had been no change. I asked her how she felt. Was her energy good? Did she have any symptoms? Was she compliant to the diet she had been given? Her reply was that she felt great, she had good energy, no symptoms, she ate really well and she did yoga on a regular basis. Other than her belly, all was good. I told her that if energy, moods and symptoms are all reflecting a happy body, there is only one place to go. Find peace with being good enough as you are. There is a core life lesson in that. The result will be either a loss of weight due to a shift in perspective (which will alter your cellular structure) or you just find peace with what is. We agreed that either way, it was a winning outcome.

Speaking to your body

The other aspect of communicating with your body flips directions. It travels from your mind to your body. What do you think about your body? What do those little voices in your head say about it? Externally, how do you speak about your body to others? How do you dress? What do you do to take care of or pamper it? In this sense we go from the receptive side of listening, to the creative control of how we choose to use our mind.

To help you shift your perspective regarding this vehicle that carries you through life, here are some musings, and ideas on strengthening this constant and precious relationship.

Create an intention that you want to have a healthy relationship with your body.

Clarifying and stating your intention, gives your brain the opportunity to look for ways that it can be fulfilled. The Reticular Activating System (RAS) is the automatic mechanism inside your brain that brings relevant information to your attention. It becomes important for creating new pathways and reaching goals because you can program it by affirming, visualizing, and practicing what you want to achieve. In essence, the more you bring conscious attention to what you want, the more the RAS is working subconsciously to attract it to you.

Consider that your body is like an infant.

It communicates through feelings and senses. Treat it with the tenderness that you would a young child. To listen to it, you need to get down to its level. You need to be willing to feel it and to act on its messages.

Be nice to your body.

Don't call it bad names and expect it to love you back. For whatever you may hate about your body, there is always something that you can find that you can love. It is all about perspective. Look for the bad and you will find it. Look for the good and you will find it. Whatever you look for, you will find.

* *

In moments of my critical stance in front of the mirror, I have been challenged by this idea of looking for what is

*beautiful. Given my own dose of 'not good enough' that I've
had to tend to, this wasn't always easy. Then I discovered my
ears. Yes, I have lovely ears. I am declaring it to the world.
They are a nice size relative to my head, the shape of the
whole ear is balanced by a firm lobe and a nicely formed inner maze. Whenever I have had any trouble with something
that I don't like, I turn to my ears for a little reminder of my
beauty. Inevitably it brings comic relief.*

**Spend time everyday in gratitude for some
aspect of your body and its capacity.**
Look below for some things that might stimulate your appreciation.

- How many miles has it walked?
- How many babies has it birthed?
- How many vocal tones can it produce?
- How many times has it sprung back from illness?
- How many times has it listened for glorious music, the sounds of birds or your children laughing?
- How many meals, snacks and binges has it digested and eliminated?
- How many feelings has it expressed through touch?
- How many times has it woken up from sleep to start a new day?
- How many gardens has it dug, homes has it renovated, jobs has it operated for?
- How often has it been available when you were ready for a soulful experience?
- How many beautiful things has it seen?
- How many wonderful meals has it tasted?
- How many different ways can it move?

- How many times has it been there for you when you weren't there for it?

**Ask not what your body can do for you,
but what you can do for your body.**
Remember JFK's famous line, "Ask not what your country can do for you, but what you can do for your country." We're just altering it a little bit to address a more personal focus. How can you pamper it?

**Throughout the day, take a moment to check in
with your body to see how it's feeling.**
Scan your body parts to see what you notice. Pay attention to its hunger, thirst, energy, mood, and symptoms. Note how you feel after each meal or snack, as well as other times of the day. Practice acting on the messages that you get.

**Dance free and wild, and/or immerse yourself in
play. Take care of your body as you go.**
Your body will feel your love and will love you back. Also practice BLMS that I introduced you to in week #7, *Take Charge of Your Emotions.*

**Try out a playful perspective where you imagine
that your body is your best friend.**
This is a friend like no other. There is not a place that you go, not a movement you make, not a breath that you take that your body isn't with you. How should you treat a lifelong friend?

Week #10

. . . .

Take Control of
Your Portions

. . .

Tackle Social Eating

Take Control of Your Portions

What you need to do

I get asked about portion sizes a lot. Most of us want clear instructions on how much we should be eating. My hope, however, is that if you followed my recommendations on recognizing your hunger in week #5, *Get in Tune with Your Hunger* and paid attention to why you are overeating in the week following, that you would find your own personal portion control. Having said that, if finding your natural hunger and satiation level is still a bit of a struggle or you just haven't practiced it enough, then you may need some straight-from-the-hip ideas about what you can do to minimize eating too much.

This week then, is about paying attention to how much you are eating and adjusting your portions by using some of the techniques mentioned here.

Why you need to do this

In a conversation about quantities of food, there is an opportunity to break a common myth – that of 'calories in, calories out'. The idea, one which we have all heard thousands of times, is that you need to burn more calories than you consume if you want to lose weight, and if you consume more than you burn, you will gain weight. This has become an accepted 'law' in the field of nutritional science. I would support that there is some truth in this – if you eat more than your body needs for fuel and raw materials, you will gain weight, but for reasons far more complex than just a simple calculation of 'calories in, calories out'. The counting of calories is an inexact science and can be misleading if used as the sole source of direction.

Calories are a measurement of the heat generated by the burning of a food. The amount of calories designated to a food is determined by energy produced when measuring it in a lab in a contraption called a 'bomb calorimeter'. Consider that how a food burns inside a device and how it is used in any person's body is not going to be the same. Only the calories from carbohydrates are used purely for energy production. In the case of protein and fats, they are used primarily as raw materials for the structures, hormones, neurotransmitters, enzymes and a variety of other basic building blocks of the body. Little of the calories of proteins and fat are used for energy production so they cannot be counted in the same way they would be in the bomb calorimeter, where they are measured purely for the production of energy.

Even if calorie counting was reliable as a single measure, I find it laughable that those who use the 'calories in, calories out' rule, rarely mention the quality of the calories. The science says that a calorie is a calorie is a calorie. Yes, inside a bomb calorimeter that may be the case. However, eating a Krispy Kreme donut that logs in at 250 calories is not going to support you to be at your ideal weight as well as 250 calories of wild caught salmon with a salad. In a donut, you have next to no protein, vitamins, minerals, fibre, and essential omega fats. You do however have lots of sugary carbs, saturated and trans fats. Which one is going to help aid your metabolic processes to burn fat better? If you can't answer that, go back to the beginning of this book and start reading again. You'll be reminded of the importance of protein for stimulating the fat-burning hormone glucagon, and how too many carbs will lead to the extra sugar being stored as fat. You will also be reminded of the importance of the good fats and the necessity to eliminate bad fats.

If the idea of calorie counting still seems like a good idea to you, consider some statistics from Health Canada. Obesity and overweight in men (ages 20 – 65) rose from 46.9% to 65.2% from 1972 to 2004 while their average caloric intake dropped across the age ranges. For women, overweight and obesity rates rose from 30.8% to 52.4% during those same years. Yet calorie consumption either dropped or remained the same.

I hope that gives you enough evidence (or at least sparks your curiosity) to consider that being in control of your portions is not about being focused only on counting your calories. Rather it is about being aware of the quality of the food that you're consuming, as well as using some techniques, ideas and visual cues to help you eat the right amounts. Augment these tips by paying attention to your body, noticing your hunger levels and you'll be on track to a way of eating that is sustainable.

How you can do this

Wait twenty minutes after eating before you go for seconds.

It takes that long for the hormones that send signals of satiation (hunger is satisfied) to catch up to your intake. You can play a game with yourself. Tell yourself that you can go for more food if in twenty minutes you still want it. See how strong your desire is then.

Get out of the kitchen.

This works particularly well if most of your cleanup is done before you sit down to eat. As soon as you are done eating, leave the kitchen to do something else that is more enticing. Go back to week #8, *Nourish Your Soul*, to establish activities that you would enjoy as much or more than eating. Make a plan to engage in those activities as soon as you are done your first plate of food.

Drink lots of water.

Often people mistake their thirst for hunger, so making sure you keep hydrated throughout the day will help with some of the overeating. Also try drinking a cup of water before each meal to create a little less room for the food.

Eat your salad before your mains.

Salad with protein is a meal in itself. Aim for it as a staple for lunch or dinner. In addition, for those meals that include other foods, eat your salad first. You are more likely to enjoy the vegetables when you are hungry than when you have already filled up on richer choices. This will intensify the love affair developing between you and your veggies. Also the fibre rich vegetables will fill in some of the space that the richer foods would take up, leading to smaller portions of the mains.

Keep the serving dishes off the table.

Best to portion out your plate at the stove or countertop and leave the extras off the table. If you have to get up and walk to get more food (rather than just reach across the table) you have a greater chance of creating a 'gap of awareness' and taking your time to determine if you really need more.

Take control of your trigger foods.

You know the foods that you have little control over. It will be easier to keep them out of your home. Then when the craving shows up, you can think before running to the store. Have those treats occasionally so you don't feel deprived (remember the 90/10 rule) but buy them in small one serving packages when you are not at home. If you must bring them into the house, divvy them up into smaller servings and store in small containers or sandwich bags. Again, this is another opportunity to create the 'gap' before you reach for more.

Eating smaller meals every 3 hours will help.

Remember that the point of eating consistently throughout the day is to stabilize hormones and blood sugar and shut down the physical cravings, so don't ignore that important rule. When you are doing that consistently, you will probably notice that you don't need to eat so much at each meal. What was once your lunch can now be divvied up into your lunch and mid-afternoon snack. Don't feel that you need to eat it all in one sitting just because it's there. As you pay more attention to your body and your level of hunger and satiation, you will get better at monitoring exactly how much you need to eat.

Divide leftovers into meal size containers.

It is easier to monitor quantities if you create single-serving sized containers of leftovers, so you can grab and go. Again if you are taking it for lunch or heating it up at the next dinner, you are less likely to eat more if the portion is contained.

When eating out, start with smaller portions.

If there is an opportunity to get a kid-sized portion, do it. Ice cream cones are always available as kiddie cones and you may realize that you are satisfied with a smaller amount. Fast food places, if you choose to go to them, also have kid-sized meals. In restaurants where there is only one adult size, pack up half of your meal before you start eating (take a container with you, or ask for a second plate or a take-home container). Learning to be assertive and ask for what you need is part of the process of taking care of yourself. Or share your meal with your dining companion.

Create a visual picture of what a reasonable portion looks like.

Stick to standard portion sizes by understanding what that looks like. Here are some metaphoric visuals to help you out:

* 4 ounces of meat or chicken is approximately the size of a hockey puck
* 2/3 cup of pasta or grains would be the size of a tennis ball
* 3/4 cup of milk or yogurt is the amount in a single serving yogurt container (175 gram size)
* 1 ounce of cheese is similar to four large dice stacked one on top of each other
* 4 ounces of fish is close to what you get in a standard size can of tuna (170 gram size – which includes the liquid)
* One serving of vegetables or fruit would be about the size of a large baseball (a softball, not a hard ball)

Take the opportunity to measure the volume with measuring cups or spoons, or the weight of food with a scale so that you can get an accurate picture. When you have done it a few times, you will get better at 'eyeballing' it. I bought my first scale only about five years ago. It has been a revelation to actually see what food weighs. It has also made it easier to follow the recipes that use weight measurements and to know how much of another food can be substituted when necessary. I highly recommend a kitchen scale for the knowledge and convenience that you'll gain from it. You don't have to spend a lot of money on one. I paid about twenty dollars for mine and it's operated well to this point, years later.

Act like a scientist with you as the research project.

Find out what it feels like to eat less food. It's an interesting exploration. Ask yourself these questions: what would it be like to eat modest amounts from a smaller plate? Would I still be hungry? How differently would I feel? Then go about exploring to see what the answers are. Creating the inquiry gives you reason to become more conscious of the process of eating and the messages that your body relays to you.

Tackle Social Eating

What you need to do

We all love to eat and to do it with others – and we certainly have lots of opportunities to do so.

Sharing good food is so delightful and pleasurable that we will continue to partake throughout our lives. Our desire to gather together to eat and drink is well entrenched in who we are as human beings. We are unlikely to escape it for any length of time. Having strategies and perspective shifts to deal with the challenge of communal eating is a crucial step to sustainable change. This week is about finding new options for handling your social life when food is involved, and taking whatever opportunities you have to practice it.

Why you need to do this

Our personal and cultural experiences are ripe with examples of food sharing. We do it to celebrate, to offer good will, to promote our status, to share in the pleasures, and as a way to spend time together. Professor Robin Fox from Rutgers University describes the powerful nature of social eating:

"It is a profoundly social urge. Food is almost always shared;
people eat together; mealtimes are events when the whole

family or settlement or village comes together. Food is also an occasion for sharing, for distributing and giving, for the expression of altruism, whether from parents to children, children to in-laws, or anyone to visitors and strangers. Food is the most important thing a mother gives a child; it is the substance of her own body, and in most parts of the world mother's milk is still the only safe food for infants. Thus food becomes not just a symbol of, but the reality of, love and security."

Due to the network of relationships, memories and beliefs, social eating can be one of the toughest areas to get a handle on. Many of us find it easy to make the right choices when we are on our own. However when we share a meal in the presence of friends, family or colleagues, more complex issues enter into the mix. There is the pure pleasure of eating with others. But we may also be caught in a web of conflict. We don't want to limit the fun, irritate or offend our hosts, or be too demanding, so we give in to others choices in order to keep harmony around the meal. We loathe being the 'party pooper.' Often, we lean heavily towards keeping the status quo and either not challenging ourselves, or those around us, to do something differently. You might recall Einstein's famous line "the definition of insanity is doing the same thing over and over again and expecting different results." Transforming your weight and your relationship with food, calls upon you to step away from your personal insanity. This means having strategies for how you party, celebrate and function at 'get-togethers.'

If you have strong inclinations towards social eating and drinking and it often gets out of control, then getting a handle on this may be one of the biggest obstacles to your sustainable success. In all likelihood, if you are reading this chapter, you have your own struggles, so I don't need to go much further in the explanation of why you need to face this challenge. Not doing it will lead to progressive weight gain over the years.

If you want to 'tackle and take down' social eating you need to eat with more awareness in social situations. Awareness comes in many forms and packages – there are different options for different situations. I describe some below. Start practicing and you will find your own mix that works for you.

How you can do it

There is no magic bullet to make you better at self-control in a social situation – but understanding some principles can go along way towards having control.

Stabilize your blood sugar.

If you go to a party, a feast or to dinner without having eaten consistently throughout the day, your blood sugar will be out of whack, your brain will be hungry for food and you won't be able to control yourself. So 'social eating principle' number one is: don't save up your calories for the end of the day so that you can indulge at the feast. That is a surefire way to being out of control. In fact, people who do that will usually eat more calories in that one meal than they would have eaten throughout the day. Eat consistently every three hours to stabilize your blood sugar, so that you're not ravenous when you get there. You may even want to consume some protein or a mini meal before you go so that you have more control. A protein shake, some cottage cheese, half a can of tuna or a leftover chicken breast with some veggies would be a perfect foil for excessive hunger and lack of control.

Improve your nutrition, up your control.

The more good nutrition you get under your belt, the more your body and taste buds will adapt to seek out higher quality of food. In other words, the healthier and closer to nature your choices are over time, the less you will be looking for the junky stuff. This will bode well at a lot of social functions because some of the foods that you would have included on your plate before will be off the list when you refine your tastes. I have a memory from about ten years ago, when I had my last donut, how unappealing and super sweet it tasted to me. I knew that it was unlikely that I would ever eat another. I grew up eating donuts and had you told me twenty years ago that I would get to a point where I would never want to eat another Timbit, I would have been skeptical.

Our taste buds adapt and our desires change. I see it in almost all of my clients who take on their health and nutrition in a committed way. It is progressive and you need to be patient because it can take years in some cases – but if you stay the course and take it a step at a time, taste bud transformation is inevitable.

The more you exercise, the less you'll want to overindulge.

This happens in part because of the reserve of endorphins, dopamine and serotonin that are providing you with good feelings and energy. The memory of those feelings can be enough to keep you from overindulging in foods and alcohol that you know will require more recovery to get you back to that pre-indulgent mood. Plus you have a close-at-hand memory of the amount of work it takes to work off the calories.

Manage your energy and you'll be better equipped to manage your willpower.

Anything that you can do to up your energy – whether it's good nutrition, more exercise, better sleep, more joy in your life, more chill-out time – the more internal energy reserves you will have. And the more internal reserves, the more willpower. Here's why: the prefrontal cortex of the brain is the location where the sensory stimulus that comes into our brain gets processed. If you are flooded with the input of a lifestyle that is constantly filled with things to do, places to go and people to see, your prefrontal cortex is using a lot of processing power to deal with that input. So what's that got to do with social eating? Well, the prefrontal cortex is also the seat of our willpower and if too much processing is being taken up by stress or overstimulation, then there isn't much left over for you to control yourself. Also providing the raw nutrients that are needed for the energy systems to work optimally plays a part in those internal reserves being available to you. So a combination of having enough quiet time and good nutrition will support greater resources of energy and more willpower.

From a psychological perspective, here are some other tidbits of awareness to take with you:

You always have a choice.

The concept that we have to eat because the hostess is providing it or because your clients or colleagues expect it, is based more on your own beliefs and cultural inclinations than it is on absolutes. The reality is, that you can choose to do whatever you want. This requires some courage as you may be pushing against the norm. Having said that, you can do it to any degree you want. You may choose to eat everything served but in far smaller quantities or to choose the most appealing dishes and excuse yourself from the rest. Or you may pre-warn your host that you have certain foods that you cannot eat at this time. These may seem like unappealing options at this point but they are doable. With practice, they get easier. Recognizing that you do have a choice is empowering. Empowerment also holds responsibility. You can no longer blame another person or the event for your social eating issues.

One of my group participants, I'll call him Jack, shared with us that his mother-in-law, who is Italian, never seemed to stop pushing him to eat more. Her food is delicious but like much of the Italian repertoire, it is loaded with carbs, lots of cheese, copious amounts of wine, and an abundance of courses. With her insistence, Jack tended to eat a lot and to gain weight every time he went to her house for a meal. He was ready to change the situation. At a group brainstorming session, it was suggested that Jack share his intentions with his in-law in a loving and non-threatening way, and be prepared for the fact that she might not like it. He agreed to the challenge. He came back from his weekend away with his spouse and Mama Maria with a renewed sense of strength. He told her, she didn't like it, but he stuck with his resolve. He left food on his plate, ate half the courses and drank only two glasses of wine. He realized that although she didn't like it, it also wasn't as big a deal as he had made it out to be. She would get over it and it ultimately it didn't seem to affect their relationship in any way that really mattered.

Be intentional and plan ahead.

There is nothing like a good plan to get you on track and keep you there. A plan can be as simple as a decision made, but the key is to do it ahead of time. Combine choice and intention and you will find yourself in a stronger, more powerful place when you arrive at your social destination. Know also that your intention should be within your reach. It needs to be doable for you.

Patty is a successful businesswoman who, along with her husband, has an active social life. Every weekend they are with friends and those gatherings are inevitably focused around food and drinks. In her challenge to lose weight, she knew that something had to change. She was clear that having five or six drinks each day was not helping her efforts. Two glasses of wine were fine but once she had a third, the alcohol contributed to a loss of control and resolve. Not having any wasn't a choice that she was willing to make, but she could drink just two glasses. I had her create a vision, seeing herself with her friends and being successful at sticking to only two glasses. It worked for her when she did it. But the practice was in doing it before every gathering. She sometimes forgot and found that her power was lessened without the intention being set.

Practice saying 'no.'

Strengthen your resolve to stay committed to your path by practicing saying 'no' in a positive way. No big drama – just tell people something simple like, "I'm prioritizing my health..." The better you get at saying 'no', the easier it will be for others to accept it. They may even be inspired by your choices and decide to join you.

Eat mindfully.

We go into the benefits of eating mindfully next week. For now, know that if you eat slowly, savouring each bite, you will give more opportunity for your satiation hormones to kick in. Once they're activated, it's much easier to stop eating. If you have trouble eating slowly, take a twenty- minute break after your first plate of food before you go for seconds. That way you give those hormones a chance to do their work. If you do decide to indulge, do it mindfully, enjoying every bite. Then get back on track at your next meal or as soon as you can.

Here are some other practical ideas to help you take charge:

- Split desserts with someone else or don't take any at all – the less sugar you get the less you will want it.

- Intersperse your alcoholic beverages with sparkling water or a sparkling/cranberry juice combo. Drink it from a wine glass or other stemware so that you still feel like you are in celebration mode and the host/hostess won't be as inclined to fill your glass with alcohol.

- Drink lots of water in between your food choices.

- Ask the restaurant server for a second plate so you can split your meal if you know it is too much for you. Or, ask the server to pack it to go.

- Get sauces and dressings on the side so you can control your consumption.

- Put foods on your plate that you can eat unlimited amounts of, such as vegetables. When it is appropriate, at a potluck or picnic, bring a vegetable dish with you to make sure you have that as an option.

- Remember your pain motivators, i.e. threats of heart disease, diabetes, abdominal cramping, etc. Bring them to mind whenever you are about to step into a social situation.

* *

A friend said to us that 'gluten makes her angry'. We laughed. The way that she said it, with a smile on her face and a twinkle in her eye, at first lead us to think that she was joking. But she wasn't. She uses 'gluten makes me angry' as a mantra to remind her that gluten grains shift her moods. She has discovered that eating them isn't worth it for her and hasn't indulged in those grains for years.

* *

Week #11

Learn to Navigate the Grocery Store

Practice Mindful Eating

Learn to Navigate the Grocery Store

What you need to do

As you become more informed about nutrition, you need to get practical about how to put that knowledge into action. This includes how you shop for food. Major decisions that affect your health and weight are made in the grocery store. If you don't know what to buy and where to find it, you will be missing the important first link in healthy meal preparation.

We tend to be loyal to our products, not necessarily because of the product themselves but because repetitive shopping is easier and faster. Consider shopping as a practice like everything else in this book. Learn what and why you need to change, and then at a pace that you can handle, alter your shopping operandi.

Make a list of what you normally buy and check it against the chart on the pages to follow to see if there would be a better substitute. Give yourself a little extra time to shop in the first few weeks of buying new foods. You will need to scout product locations, do some comparisons and read labels. When you have figured out what to buy after a few times of traveling through the store, your pathway and choices will become automated and you'll be able to whip through your shopping as fast as ever. This week's info is companion material to week #4, *Eat Close to Nature*. This time we take it a little further into the practical aspects of shopping.

Why you need to this

It is important for every consumer to understand a basic premise about the food industry – it is not health that drives it. The bottom line is economics. Like most other industries, there are some major players (Coca Cola, Kraft, General Mills are a few familiar names) that are publicly traded and need to increase their profit margins every quarter. How do they do that? By selling us more food or by making it cheaper. Usually it's both.

Supermarkets are designed down to the detail, based on multitudes of studies and years of research on what gets consumers to spend more money in their stores. Social scientists are hired to research people's buying habits and preferences. Neuroscientists enlighten the industry on how to influence us based on the workings of our brain. Market analysts videotape us to see how we move through the aisles and how to position products accordingly. One principle is well entrenched in supermarket science: the more visible a product is, the better it will sell. Professor of nutrition and author of *What to Eat*, Marion Nestle suggests an interesting concept. "Think of the supermarket as a particularly intense real estate market in which every product competes fiercely against every other for precious space. Because you can see products most easily at eye level, at the ends of aisles, and at the checkout counters, these areas are prime real estate."

Determining what you see most and thus are more likely to buy is not based on the science of good nutrition but on who has the deepest pockets to pay for the incentives and the advertising that goes along with the preferred product placement.

Barry is a province-wide rep for an artisan bread company out of Montreal. He has taken samples of his bread to all of the major high-end grocers in the city and had them test the bread for quality of flavour, texture and next day freshness. Nine out of ten times the grocers have preferred it to any other artisan bread that they carry, including the major competitor who is now owned by the parent company of the biggest grocery store chain in the country. Despite

the recognition that they could provide a superior product
to their customers, Barry's smaller company has not been
able to compete with the incentive demands that the grocers
require to feature his product. The competitor still rules be-
cause they are willing and able to pay big money to remain
king of the bread department.

Barry's experience is just one tiny example of an industry that is ripe with underhanded dealings that ultimately drives the products that you're exposed to. If a high profit can be made from a particular type and brand, then you can guarantee that you will see more of it. Consider that some of the highest grossing grocery product sales are soft drinks, boxed cereals, and frozen dinners. Next time you're in the grocery store notice the amount of space dedicated to those categories. These are major profit items. Even if the profit margins were not great, the 'slotting fees' that the companies pay for the prime locations make up for it. Unfortunately, the fact that these foods lack nutritional value seems an irrelevant point for the bottom line.

Before you even walk into the grocery store you have witnessed innumerable commercials and advertisements, online and in print, whose sole purpose is to entice you to try a food, with the hopes that you will develop brand loyalty to that particular food or drink. As a health conscious consumer, it's likely that you have paid attention to the products that claim to love your heart, lower cholesterol, increase your fibre, eliminate trans fats, improve your digestive health and help you lose weight. The marketing is designed to draw your attention to the terms that imply wellness – phytosterols, probiotics, heart check, natural, whole grains. At the same time, the intention is to also distract you from the fact that these supposedly healthy products are overly processed, often containing high amounts of fat, sugar, and salt, or chemicals that substitute for the lack of one or more of fat, sugar and salt.

In his book, *The End of Overeating*, Dr. David Kessler lays out a case for the ingenious ways that the industry succeeds in getting you to like their food. He talks about a study that was sponsored by McCormick. Called 'Crave-It!', it asked several thousand people questions about twenty-one categories of food. Jacqueline Beckley, head of a product development group and co-designer of the study, stated, "My intention was to unlock the code of craveability". Craveability refers to the irresistibility of a food, the level of comfort it provides, and your desire to return to it over and over again. From Kessler's book: "Based on its collected data, the Crave-It! study sorted respondents into three groups: the classics, the variety seekers, and the imaginers. Later they added a fourth group, those who focus on good nutrition. People with a classic mind-set crave highly familiar standards, while variety seekers look for novelty (this is the population for whom the industry designs new flavors of potato chips). "The imaginers," said Beckley, "are driven by ambience or romance or emotionality. It is not about the food but about the concept of food."

The industry knows who they are marketing to when they set out to sell their products. Think of Coca Cola. The original Coke is there for the classic cravers, and more than one hundred choices in Coca Cola freestyle offers enough for the variety seekers. For the imaginers, the 'open happiness' campaign and any of the quite brilliant Coke commercials – the polar bears, Move to the Beat, the happiness truck – are an appeal to them. And for the nutritionally conscious, Coke Zero, with zero calories might be guilt-free enough to convince them to buy. Appealing to the healthy mindset a little further, there is an ad campaign that distracts attention away from the lack of nutrition in any soft drink, focusing your attention instead on sponsoring a physical activity campaign for greater fitness. It implies a focus on health without actually offering it (at least in their own products). Don't get me wrong. There's nothing wrong with supporting more exercise for the masses and especially for kids whose activity levels have declined in the past two decades. But it's crucial to your own health to be able to dissect the emotions that might be triggered by marketing. Be clear that your wellbeing will not come from a bottle of pop, no matter how many calories it doesn't have.

You may wonder why there aren't more regulations to hold companies and stores accountable to the quality of food that consumers are exposed to. Unfortunately, the government, medical industry, and associations who are supposed to be educating and protecting us, are constantly lobbied to by the industry players. Money rules. The food industry big boys promise funding and support to those who support them. An example is the funding that is given to the Canadian Foundation for Dietetic Research.

Dieticians are supposedly setting the standards for good nutrition at the level of government and public health. Yet, take a look at who is, in part, funding their research.

- Dairy Farmers of Canada
- Nestle Healthcare Nutrition
- The Centrum Foundation and Wyeth Consumer Health Care Inc.
- Campbell's Food Service and Campbell Company of Canada
- Kraft Canada Ltd.
- McCain Foods (Canada)
- McDonald's Restaurants of Canada Limited
- Compass Group Canada
- Unilever Canada Inc. (Becel, Slim-Fast, Ben & Jerry's, Lipton, Knorr, etc)
- Abbott Nutrition Canada (Ensure, Similac, etc.)
- Almond Board of Canada
- ARAMARK Canada Ltd.
- Canola Council of Canada
- Egg Farmers of Canada
- General Mills Canada Corporation
- Kellogg Canada Inc.
- Loblaw Companies Ltd
- Mead Johnson Nutrition (Enfamil, etc)
- PepsiCo Canada

Are the companies who are producing highly manufactured products of convenience the ones that should be influencing those who set the standards for optimal health?

(The Academy of Nutrition and Dietetics, the American branch of the dietician's association has funding from many of the same donors.)

How you can do it

The bottom line of grocery store navigation is that you can't trust the food industry that is marketing to you as your source of information for what is healthy. You have to be a critical thinker and an objective shopper. You'll have to stay alert through every level that you are marketed to, from the advertisements that you see in the media, to where you shop, to what you throw in your cart as you maneuver your way through the booby-trapped aisles.

Here are some thoughts to help you do that.

Plan ahead.

Knowing what meals you want to prepare for the week will take the guess work out of shopping and prep time. It will ensure that you have everything available as needed and will cut down on desperate food consumption.

Make a list.

You will save time, money, and your health, by sticking to your plan and making a list before you go. Supermarket design science knows you will buy more, the more time you are there and the more products you see. So be clear about what you need when you enter and stick to your list.

Eat before shopping.

Temptations are greater when you are hungry. Make sure to stabilize your blood sugar by eating before you go, including some protein and fibre in that pre-shopping meal.

Shop the periphery of the store.

The outside aisles are where you will find the unprocessed foods – vegetables, fruit, dairy, fish, meats and foods that require refrigeration. These are the foods that are closer to nature, less processed and higher in nutrition.

Be cautious of brands that have marketing campaigns.

Be extra cautious if they are marketing some health claim. Chances are they have found one isolated substance that is a 'buzz' word, like 'Omega 3', 'active bacterial culture' or 'phytosterols' and they are including it along with a bunch of other cheap ingredients. They assume that as an uneducated consumer you will buy into the health claim. Also, the bigger the campaign, the larger the percentage of their cost is going towards marketing and less is going towards making a good quality food.

Read the label, looking for ingredients that you don't understand.

When you find them, don't buy it. If it says modified anything, do you know what it is? Do you know what 'High Fructose Corn Syrup' is? Do you know what BHT is? Even innocuous substances that are just synthetic vitamins and minerals are a note to be cautious, because if they are adding them back in, there is little nutrition left from the actual substance.

When it comes to numbers such as grams of fat or carbohydrates, don't get too hung up on them, as the quality of what you are eating matters more. However if you want a guideline, besides looking for foods that are minimally processed, ideally it should have low levels of sodium (below 480 mg/ serving), sugar (less than 5 gm/serving), and no hydrogenated or trans fats.

Make treats a treat.

Having what you love once in a while is an important component of sustainability. Remember the principle of 90/10. One of the ways to honor that is to make your treat time a special occasion rather than a constant. Buying a package of cookies makes them readily available for anytime that you want them – which if you are like most people, will be daily. However buying one cookie, allows you the one treat and creates space so that you can deal with cravings in healthier ways. Optionally make your treat time an adventure. For example, go for a walk for an ice cream cone. If there is one a block away and a better one, ten blocks away, take the longer trip. Also when you get there, remember to check in with yourself – can you be satisfied with one scoop, rather than two or three?

Beyond these general recommendations, there is a lot to know about the hazards of shopping, so much so that it could be a book in itself. However I have included a simple guide below that will offer some support. If you are still not sure about something, go back to the basics and keep it close to nature. And remember, if you look for the convenience of packaged foods, it comes at a cost. It is not as nutritionally dense and is likely to have cheap substances that will wreck havoc on your metabolism.

Note: As mentioned in Week #2, *Eat Close to Nature*, eating organic and as natural as possible costs more money. If this is not doable for you, don't fret it. Do what you can and use the guidelines below to look for products that have fewer ingredients that you don't know. If I mention organic, raw or pasture-raised and you can't find it or afford it, do your best to just get it closer to its natural form.

Food	Look for	Be cautious of
Yogurt	organic (preferably) milk and bacterial culture traditionally made, cheesecloth strained Greek yogurt for its higher protein content go for plain plus fresh fruit	health claims incl. having an exclusive probiotic bacteria chemical sweeteners and additives, high sugar content ultra-filtration which denatures the whey proteins added milk protein concentrates
Milk, butter	organic or pasture-raised milk goats milk alternative non-dairy options	commercially farmed dairy all milk if you have respiratory or digestive issues
Cheese	organic or raw natural cheeses goat and sheep cheese	processed cheese slices and spreads orange cheese is colored with annato which people can be allergic to
Whipping cream, ice cream	real whipping cream, use moderately choose real ice cream with milk, cream, sugar, natural flavorings sorbet or gelato all to be seen as a treat occasionally	whipped dessert toppings and ice cream is likely to contain additives, high fructose corn syrup, hydrogenated or other toxic fats, modified milk ingredients, artificial flavorings, chemical sweeteners low fat will mean higher additives and sugar to make up for lack of fat content

Food	Look for	Be cautious of
Non-dairy beverages	almond, hemp or rice milk preferably unsweetened	high sugar content soy milk which can cause allergic reactions, also cause digestive or thyroid issues in some
Coffee whitener or creamer	organic milk or cream	avoid artificial whiteners and creamers due to toxic fats and additives
Margarine, Non-dairy spreads	Earth Balance spreads coconut oil pestos	be particularly cautious of health claims of margarines – this is a cheaply made, highly manufactured food with the risk of cancer-causing poly-aromatic hydrocarbons
Cooking oils	dark, glass bottles oils that are cold pressed – avocado and coconut oils for cooking, olive oil for adding to foods	mass produced oils in clear bottles, esp. clear plastic vegetable, corn, canola oils when using large tins, check to see whether their oil in bottles is in dark glass cooking sprays
Salad dressing	olive oil or other quality oils of choice balsamic, white wine or other vinegars or lemon juice herbs, spices, Celtic or Himalayan sea salt, fresh pepper	commercial salad dressings due to poor quality fats, sugar and chemical additives
Eggs, Chicken	pasture raised organic	commercially raised chickens and eggs from them – they are inhumanely raised and under too much stress which affects the quality of the eggs and meat free run or free range means they are out of cages but still trapped on the factory floor, better choice but still not great Omega 3 eggs just means that flax has been added to their feed – they are still inhumanely raised

Food	Look for	Be cautious of
Meat	pasture raised – the meat will have a better fat profile and will contain less stress hormones organic extra lean ground turkey, beef or veggie patties as alternative to frozen beef patties fresh oven roasted sliced turkey or chicken breast	meat from commercially raised animals due to inhumane practices, high stress hormone content and higher saturated fat profiles packaged deli meats that have high nitrate content (or cultured celery extract) wieners, sausages, luncheon meat, corned beef keep meat consumption, even pasture or organic, moderate due to high fat profiles and drain on environmental resources
Fish	Arctic char canned light or Yellowfin tuna * US /Canadian Pacific Albacore* fish canned in water wild Alaskan salmon Alaskan or Pacific halibut Alaskan or BC sablefish farmed rainbow trout US farmed tilapia mackerel anchovies Pacific sardines farmed oysters, not wild US haddock farmed mussels**	shark or swordfish kingfish or marlin Chilean sea bass fresh or frozen tuna, Asian Albacore, Bluefin, Bigeye tuna fish canned in oil farmed Atlantic salmon Atlantic and Pacific cod (if not from Alaska) Atlantic halibut walleye, perch Asian tilapia mahi mahi, international rockfish or Pacific snapper monkfish farmed shrimp, except from the US and Canada orange roughy**
Vegetables and Fruit	locally grown or organic, ideally both if local or organic is not possible, all are acceptable frozen is a good alternative for convenience small producer of sprouts	wilted, bruised, under-ripe, over-ripe, too soft (for those that should be hard) canned, although if you must, get in its own juice french fries commercial sprouts due to molds

Food	Look for	Be cautious of
Bread	stone ground whole grains artisan breads, sourdough cultures Organic grains – rye, spelt, kamut rice, bean or potato flours for gluten intolerance yeast-free for digestive issues	big company brands that include poor quality fats, additives and preservatives commercial wheat-based breads (commercialization has altered the original grain) white bread
Cereals	oatmeal or other whole grain hot cereals muesli, some granola Chia Wonder Cereal (recipe at www.foodcoach.ca) 7 g sugar or less, 4 g of fibre or more, 4 g of protein or more per serving	most commercial cereals, as they are highly processed with loads of sugar and bad fats watch out for health claims, read the nutrition labels instead, looking for ingredients that you don't recognize and the sugar, fibre and protein content
Crackers	low fat whole grain crackers with ingredients that you recognize gluten free crackers brown rice cakes (unsalted or lightly salted)	most commercial crackers, as they are highly processed with lots of salt and bad fats watch out for health claims, read the nutrition labels instead looking for ingredients that you don't recognize and the salt, sugar, fibre content
Pasta, noodles, macaroni	organic whole wheat, wild or brown rice or ancient grain pastas gluten free pastas fresh homemade pasta Udon or soba noodles made partially from buckwheat	fried instant Asian noodles boxed macaroni excessive amounts of wheat pasta due to the alteration of wheat crops
Baked products	whole grain flours – spelt, oats, organic whole wheat, rice (to make your own from scratch), home bake to have control over ingredients gluten free minimum 4 g of fibre use fresh and dried fruit	commercially baked products, store bought muffins, cakes and pies – high in poor quality fats, sugar, additives, wheat, likely contains toxic fats, low in nutrients ready-to-bake mixes

Food	Look for	Be cautious of
Snacks	plain popcorn	potato chips, corn chips
	fresh and dried fruits, raw nuts and seeds	flavoured microwave popcorn
	pure dark chocolate, min 70% cacao for maximum antioxidants	fruit bars
		candies, chocolate bars
	baked potato or tortilla chips	gum
Beverages	water – distilled, reverse osmosis, spring, tap, sparkling in moderation	soft drinks – high in sugar, chemical sweeteners/additives, high fructose corn syrup, artificial flavourings, caffeine
	lemon water	flavoured waters
	herbal teas, preferably from loose leaf	
	fresh squeezed fruit and vegetable juices (drink within 20 minutes of juicing)	minimize commercial fruit juice due to high sugar, low nutrient content
	coconut water	fruit drinks due to high sugar and artificial flavours
	coffee from freshly roasted, freshly ground beans	sweetened drink mixes

* For recommended tuna intakes dependent on age, consult my blog, Which fish are health to eat? at www.foodcoach.ca

** fish and seafood listings from the sustainable seafood site, www.seachoice.org or in the US www.seawatch.org . These have more comprehensive lists than I could include here and they are changeable, dependent on environmental conditions. It is advisable to consult their site on a regular basis to see updates on health and environmental concerns for fish and seafood.

Practice Mindful Eating

What you need to do

How often have you finished a meal and realized that you barely tasted it? Or that you ate it on the run, in a state of tension, or consumed it along with a gulp or two of guilt? When you have eaten like that, did you feel satisfied?

Compare that to one of your great food memories. Think about the sensuality of that experience, the flavours, textures, the company and surroundings. It is far more likely that your good food memories were ones that you were fully present to. You probably weren't on the computer, watching TV or driving while you were eating.

You might see multi-tasking as a necessity due to your busy life. You might even take pride in your capacity to do it. And yes, our brains do have the ability to process thousands of bits of information at a time. Our minds however, can fully focus on only one event in any given moment. Although it seems like you have an adept capacity to breathe, talk on the phone, make dinner, and point directions to your children all at once, to give attention to one activity means occluding full awareness of another.

Therefore if we apply multi-tasking to mealtime, if you are focused on other things while you eat, you are not going to notice what is just about to go down your gullet. Distracted eating sets the stage for mindless mouth filling, in which we come to the end of our meal and wonder where it went and why we are not satisfied.

Satisfaction it seems, plays a greater importance in the big picture of weight loss than any proponents of dieting would have previously lead you to believe. It takes us beyond nutrition as purely a material science, grounded in molecules of protein, fat, carbohydrate, vitamins, minerals, enzymes and water. Satisfaction brings nourishment into the picture. Nourishment can be likened to the *heart* or the *art* of nutrition, the feeding of not only your body, but also your mind and soul.

My partner Barry and I took some classes in tantric yoga, which is a practice that is dependent on being present. In one of those classes, we spent at least fifteen minutes taking our time to explore, and eventually eat a single raisin. It required an engagement of all of the senses, and the reward was the most luscious raisin that I have ever eaten. It amazed me how many different hues and textures that I could see as I held that raisin up to the light, how it felt in my mouth and finally when I was able to burst it open to expose its juicy sweetness, how rich in flavor it was. How can a single raisin be so nourishing? My mind was fully engaged in the experience rather than being distracted. The result was to turn up the volume on my senses.

Compare that to the full plate of salad that I ate a few nights later, as I was rushing to get to a 7:00 meeting. Was I fully awake, fully present to that experience? No. I could feel that my body was in an anxious state. My mind was halfway out the door. I couldn't tell you anything about the flavors, textures or delight of eating that salad. Being nourished was

*dependent on my presence, not on the salad's capacity to
provide nutrition, which it does by the handful.*

Imagine how much more sustainable the entire weight loss process would
be if you had deeper levels of satisfaction and your entire being felt nourished. Nourishment depends on mindfulness.

Mindfulness is about "being present in the moment in a non-judgmental
way". The dictionary on my computer defines it as "a mental state achieved
by focusing one's awareness on the present moment, while calmly acknowl-
edging and accepting one's feelings, thoughts, and bodily sensations."

This week then, is about mindful eating – what it is, why your vitality depends on it, how being mindful will make a difference to your weight and
how you can do it. Have fun. Take pleasure.

Why you need to do it

The 'how' of eating may be as important as the 'what', 'when', and 'why'.
If you eat with a negative state of mind, you will absorb less of the nutrients than if you were to eat in a positive and relaxed state. Emotional
tension, guilt, or stress, triggers the hypothalamus of the brain to turn up
the volume of the sympathetic nervous system (SNS) that regulates your
stress response. Under stress, there is less blood flow and oxygen sent to
the gut, nutrient absorption slows down, and stored nutrients get excreted
at a faster rate. Thyroid hormones, serotonin, testosterone and DHEA –
important hormones for fat metabolism – decrease in production. At the
same time that the SNS turns up its emissions, the hypothalamus tells the
opposing parasympathetic nervous system (PNS) to turn down its output.
Now, guess which side of the nervous system turns on our full digestive
power? Yes, the PNS. Since digestion is ruled primarily by the parasympathetic system, not only will you miss out on being present to the pleasures
of eating that are enhanced by relaxation, you also won't receive the full
nutritional value of what you're eating.

There is a connection between tasting a food, pleasure and metabolism.
'Cephalic phase digestive response' is a mind-centered hormonal response

to the sensuality of eating. This brain-initiated response triggers the flow of digestive juices and enzymes to ready our body for incoming foods. Cephalic, meaning 'of the head', is stimulated by our attention to the visual, aromatic, environmental and the taste qualities of our eating experience. Without this awareness, we will lose part of our digestive power, as well as some of our thermogenic ability. Thermogenesis is the body's capacity to generate heat, in essence, to burn calories.

During the eighties, two researchers from Laval University in Montreal studied the effects of the cephalic phase on thermogenesis. In two separate studies, their human subjects demonstrated that heat generation was increased by their sensory experience of the food. In one, they compared a meal eaten normally to one that was fed to them through a gastric tube to bypass the taste, visuals and aromas. When ingested orally, there was a three-fold increase in thermogenesis within fifteen minutes of eating. Whereas tube feeding reduced their heat production by four times. In the other study, they compared one meal, eaten normally, to another where the subjects had to spit out their food after chewing it. In this case they engaged the cephalic phase experience but they did not actually consume anything. Amazingly, the overall thermogenic effect in the hour following the meal, was the same whether they ingested it or not.

Although it is unclear about how big a role cephalic phase responses play in digestion, it is apparent that our capacity to make full use of the nutrients, to metabolize our food and produce energy is dependent on being present to the sensory qualities of what we consume. This is where mindfulness plays a role.

Mindfulness affects the satisfaction of our meal in two ways: by reducing distractions and by increasing attentiveness. Each factors into the satisfaction that we feel on completion of the meal and the likelihood or not, of eating more later.

In a study published in the American Journal of Clinical Nutrition in 2011, forty-four people were broken into two groups, one who ate their lunch while playing a game of solitaire on the computer and another, who ate the same meal without distractions. The distracted individuals felt less full after their lunch, and in a taste test thirty minutes following lunch, they ate one hundred percent more biscuits than the non-distracted individuals.

They also had significantly less memory recall of their meal than those who ate without distraction.

In another study, twenty-nine female subjects were placed into three groups: one that was mindful while they ate, focusing on the sensual qualities of the food (the food focus group). Another group was given the task of reading a newspaper article about food while eating (the food thoughts group). The third group was given no secondary task to do while they ate (neutral control group). They rated the participants on vividness of memory of the meal, as well as on their cookie intake later that afternoon. In the food focus group, they had less appetite before the snack session, they ate significantly less cookies and their memory was vividly higher than the other two groups. Researchers Higgs and Donohue concluded, "These results suggest that enhancing meal memory by paying attention to food while eating can reduce later intake and are consistent with the suggestion that memory plays an important role in appetite control."

I would guess that you can relate to this from personal experience. Go back to the questions that I asked you before, about meals that you've eaten on the run and ones that you can remember as being a great experience. Did one produce more satisfaction and a sense of being nourished than the other?

One of my great food experiences took place at a local restaurant. I ordered a dessert, a flourless chocolate torte, served slightly warmed with homemade roasted banana ice cream. I ate it slowly, savouring every mouthful. The combination of warm and cold, creamy and firm, not too sweet yet rich, was to die for!! All the factors were in place for that dessert to be fully satisfying. I was with good company, we had had lots of laughs and great conversation, and the room was warm, inviting, and calm. I had preceded the dessert with a light and beautifully presented main course. I was fully present and had space in my belly. How different

that same dessert would be if we took it to go in a Styrofoam
container, ate it while we watched the evening news and felt
guilty for devouring it so late when we really didn't need it.

Being mindful around food allows you to discover more about what your hunger and satiation feel like, and gives you room to respond to your body's needs in an appropriate way. Tailoring your food intake to an ideal that is personalized for you demands this type of attention. It also offers you the foundation to include your favourite indulgences in your diet because the satiation hormones will kick in faster to tell you when you have had enough.

The implications for mindfulness go beyond just how much and what type of food you eat. Being present lays the foundation for a deeper sense of satisfaction with your life, for an enhanced sense of being nourished. The practice doesn't need to begin or end with eating. Mindfulness can be applied in any aspect of your daily activities. The more you do it, the better you'll get at it. And the effects of being mindful in one way will generate presence in others. So take the challenge. Do it when you eat. Do it when you're exercising or when you're out for a walk. Do it anywhere, anytime.

How you can do it

Below you will find exercises to stimulate mindful eating. But you needn't limit your mindfulness to your eating experiences. Practice it in other areas of your life and you will find it easier to do when you are eating. For example, pick a quality that you want to pay attention to while you go through your day, such as beauty, uniqueness, calm. Then pay attention. Whatever you choose to look for, you will find it. This of course, applies to negative qualities as well. How you focus your mind is a choice and a practice. You will build your mind muscle as you train it.

There is this wonderful part of the brain, that I mentioned previously, called the Reticular Activating System (RAS) that supports your ability to do this. Choosing to become mindful about something will stimulate the RAS to make it easier for you to notice it. It does this by bringing relevant information to your attention. As an example, in the experiences of mindful eating, the RAS is turning up your senses towards the food in front of you to enhance your attention. Whatever you decide to focus your attention on, the RAS will help you notice more of it and to notice it more intensely.

A young client who had not grown up eating a lot of vegetables, wanted to include more of them in her diet. Her repertoire to that point had included the standards: cucumber, iceberg lettuce, tomato, peppers, peas and carrots. Every couple weeks, she chose a new vegetable to get to know. She started with broccoli, and then moved onto romaine lettuce, kale, cauliflower, fennel, radicchio, sweet potato and squash. She discovered this world of vegetables that she had never noticed before. Recipes started coming to her from friends. She would turn on the food channel to find shows focused on a vegetable she was exploring. She began noticing vegetables from other countries that she didn't know existed. Because she made it important, her mind supported her efforts to broaden her vegetable horizons.

The RAS helps you narrow your focus towards your priorities. When it comes to eating mindfully this is helpful, because without it, the process of eating can be boring. Reading a good magazine while eating can be much more interesting. Eating is so well practiced, there is not much new about it to hold our attention, so we need to have something that we focus on to enhance the pleasure.

Pavel Somov, PhD, author of *Eating the Moment* says it well. "As soon as we see food, we know what to expect taste-wise. And as soon as we know what to expect, we stop paying attention. This makes sense: the mind is a kind of curmudgeon that doesn't like to waste its attention span on anything that it already knows. Unfortunately, this is how we shortchange our eating experience."

Enhancing the sensual and pleasurable qualities of your meal can be both fun and mindful. Here are a few ideas that you can experiment with to see how much your level of satisfaction increases:

- Slow down and chew your food more, and when you do so pay attention to where in your mouth you experience the greatest taste sensations.
- Include a minimum of three different colors on your plate. Then count how many textures you can see.
- Add candles to the table and turn the lights down low.
- Eat outside beside a garden, or go on a picnic.
- Take the time to do ten (or at least five) deep breaths before you pick up your fork.
- Say a blessing or sing a song before eating.
- Go for a walk between preparing a meal and sitting down to eat it.
- Inhale the aromas of your food to involve the pleasure of your olfactory sense, which is so closely tied to taste sensations.
- Ask your belly what it wants and follow that.
- Put on beautiful relaxing music to accompany your dinner.

If you want to take this a little further, here are a few exercises to stimulate the practice of eating mindfully.

Breathing

The simplest exercise and one that you can do any and every time you eat (you may not, but you could), is to take ten deep breaths just before you dig into your food. Smell your food while you do it. This will shift you into parasympathetic dominance, the part of your nervous system that I mentioned before that turns on relaxation and strengthens your digestion. Breathing is the quickest way to move into a powerful digestive state and to bring you into a connection with your food.

Distraction-Free Eating

Choose a meal that is consistently eaten with the most distraction – eating dinner in front of a favorite TV show, eating an afternoon snack while driving, eating lunch while surfing the net, a late night snack while reading in bed – and choose one or two times per week in which you will eat that meal without any distractions. Instead you will focus on the eating experience.

The Four Aspects of Taste

Focus your attention on discovering which of the four taste sensations – sweet, salty, sour, bitter – or combinations thereof, are in your food. There are obvious ones: cookies are sweet, chips are salty, lemon is sour, and radicchio is bitter. But do you enjoy the subtler qualities that can be found in natural foods? For example, the sweetness in bell peppers? The saltiness in celery? The sourness in yogurt and the bitterness of kale? You can also use the four tastes to identify different types of the same food, much like a connoisseur of wine, beer or coffee will notice the subtle changes in flavor and aroma. Try it with various brands of dark chocolate, cheese or apples.

Developing a vocabulary for texture

The mind needs categories to be able to develop a subtler awareness of texture. What kind of mouth-feel does this food have? Is it watery, airy, creamy, tough, soft, crumbly, crunchy, silky, chewy, crackly, flaky, stringy, grainy, spongy, oily, drying, cooling, irritating, or spicy?

Are there one or more textures that you prefer? Don't fancy as much?

Here are some foods that offer a good testing ground for practicing your texture vocabulary:

- Pomegranate
- Lychee
- Parsley
- Hard boiled egg
- Cheese
- Sauerkraut (drain the liquid)

- Citrus slices (grapefruit, mandarin, orange)
- Asparagus
- Olives
- Strawberries
- Cherries
- Chocolate

These suggestions are offered as a starting point. Any food can be eaten mindfully. In doing so, you will discover more about it.

Savouring the Raisin

This is the exercise that Barry and I first did in a tantra class. I now do it in my own workshops because it is such fun to do in a group. In one of those workshops, during the discussion following this exercise (where we used a square of dark chocolate instead of a raisin), a man I'll call Greg shared his experience.

Greg is a man in his sixties, in good health, retired from an impressive career as a businessman, a world traveler. I mention this only to note that he has had a lot of life experience. Yet his comment after this exercise, was "This has just changed my life." I asked him what he meant by that. "I have never been able to eat a piece of chocolate slowly or with so much focus. Nor have I ever gotten so much pleasure from it. Usually, I gorge down chocolate. I will remember what has just happened here." I see Greg every year at the creativity conference where I lead this workshop. In the years following that first experience, he has continued to remind me of the impact that it has had on his life in how he eats, and the awareness of his senses. This simple fifteen-minute exercise wields a lot of power.

Although the group experience enhances its affect, I also give this exercise to individual clients as homework.

Choose one plump, juicy raisin or one small square of chocolate to do this exercise. If you don't like either, choose some other small food item that you do like – a date, fig, almond, mandarin section, or something else. If your food item isn't wrapped in its own packaging, then place it in a clear sandwich bag.

Find a place to sit where you can be quiet and without distractions for 10 – 15 minutes.

Focus on deep breathing to still your mind and to become more present in your body.

Now bring your attention to that delightful little morsel in front of you.

- Spend some time admiring the raisin (or other) as it rests in its little bag. Hold it up to the light to observe its hues and textures. Feel its shape as you roll it inside its plastic casing. Spend at least two minutes in this stage.
- Now you can remove it from its bag. Can you feel the anticipation grow as you open the bag, before it drops into your hand?
- Use your vision to admire its texture, its shape, its hues.
- Feel how it rolls between your fingers and on your hand.
- Squeeze it, mold it.
- Roll it around your face and across your lips.
- Smell it.
- Don't rush your pleasure. There is no place more important to be than right here with this raisin.
- Hold the raisin between your lips. Let your tongue taste its sweetness.
- Let it slide into the front of your mouth. Suck on it. Roll it. Squeeze it. Breathe it in.
- Bring your teeth into play but do not bite it fully yet.

- Taste the juices as you begin to break its skin with your front teeth.

- Feel all around it with your tongue.

- Now slowly begin to chew it, letting the juice fill your mouth with its flavor.

- Chew it until it is like liquid and then feel it slide down your throat.

Blind Taste-Testing (do this alone or with a partner)

This one takes a little more setup but it's worth it. From my experience, everyone should have 'eating blindfolded' on the bucket-list of things to do at least once in their lifetime, if not on a semi-regular basis. This is an incredibly sensual experience. It's more fun with a partner but it can be done alone as well. It is also an exercise that I do in my workshops. It is often one of the highlights of the day.

- Choose some simple foods that you can pick up easily with your fingers (if you are working alone) or that can be easily handled with a fork (if you are working with a partner) and lay them out on a plate in front of you. Choose foods of different textures and inclusive of the different tastes of sweet, salty, sour, bitter. As a starting point, six different foods, one mouthful of each, is a good amount.

- Put a blindfold on yourself, making sure that you can't peek out to see what's coming.

- Let your partner choose which food to feed to you, so that it is a surprise. If you are on your own, reach down to pick up what is on your plate, allowing whatever your fingers touch first to become your next food. But it is crucial to take your time. Let anticipation grow.

- Notice the aroma as it gets closer to your face. (When vision is out of the mix, the olfactory sense becomes heightened).

- As it gets nearer your mouth, let your partner (or yourself) feed you slowly, touching it to your lips, moving it under your nose, letting your tongue have a taste but not yet putting it into your mouth.

- Then once it is in your mouth, chew it slowly, paying attention to its texture, juices, flavours.

Describe your experience to your partner either during or after the exercise. If working alone, I would suggest that you write down what you experienced.

Week #12

· · · · · · · · · · · · · · · ·

Consider Researched
Supplements

· · ·

Set Up Your Environment
for Success

Consider Researched Supplements

What you need to do

The magic pill in the little bottle that's going to make your fat melt away is an enticing prospect, so enticing that the weight loss industry pulls in around three billion a year in the U.S. alone on retail and multi-level weight loss products. Market Research News estimates that the global market for weight loss nutraceuticals in 2014 will be $350 billion US. The reality is that weight loss supplements mostly just fuel a population that's desperate to lose weight and to do it quickly, without working to change their lifestyle. Over the years, I have witnessed this desperation.

For ten years, I worked as a nutritional advisor in Canada's largest supplement store, one that is well known for its professional staff and hard-to-get products. One mention of a product by Dr. Oz was enough for people to blindly leap with enthusiasm for us to take their money, completely ignoring any suggestions that it may not be the answer they're looking for. Case in point was when he talked about raspberry ketones being "the number one miracle in a bottle to burn your fat." When this particular show was aired in the spring of 2012, there was only one study done with rats and a couple in test tubes. (This hardly constitutes 'a miracle in a bottle.') Within two days we had over 150 people on a special order list after our supply of the product was sold out. I have only seen that kind of frenzy once before and that was for another weight loss product.

(Just to be clear, I think that Dr. Oz is doing a great job of informing a mass audience of alternative routes to health. However it's important to bear in mind that he is in the entertainment business as much as he is in the health field. Entertainment comes with its own brand of sensationalism and drama.)

I suspect that if you are reading this book, you have already accepted, possibly with more than a little resistance, that there is nothing you can 'take' that will do the work for you. Having said that, there is some help to be gleaned from quality supplementation, focused on your particular needs, taken at the right time and for the right reasons. I'm here to give you what I think is a balanced perspective on weight loss supplements. This comes from my years of working as an advisor in the supplement industry, being exposed to numerous multi-level companies, working with hundreds of clients and weekly reviews of published research.

This week then, is offered to you first and foremost, as an information overview – secondly, as an opportunity to add in the support of supplements if it seems appropriate to do so.

Why you need to do this

Let's talk about supplements in general first. It's possible that you may not need to take them at all, especially if you have jumped on board the close-to-nature, well-balanced, no-manufactured-food bandwagon and your health and weight have reached optimal levels. However, most people still have room to improve when it comes to their food choices. High stress, air pollution, mineral-depleted soil, compromised water supplies and of course food manufacturing, storage and transport all play a role in a higher demand for nutrients that we would have gotten naturally from our 'food-scape.' And when it comes to the healing of long-standing health issues, you can wait a long time to see therapeutic results from food alone. Having said that, nothing you can take in a bottle will ever replace the value of eating well. Rather, supplements are there to catalyze the beneficial effects of nutrient-dense food. They also act as a kind of insurance, to help minimize sickness down the road.

In my clinical practice, I never recommend weight loss products until someone is on solid ground with a healthy diet; and even then, only occasionally. My reasons? Mostly, I am focused on supporting the underlying issues that are interfering with a person's metabolism and wellbeing. For a look at what those issues could be, go to the addendum, *10 Physical Issues that will Stop You from Losing Weight (Despite Your Best Efforts)*. Outside of clinical support, there is some hope to be had in the form of weight loss supplements but I suggest caution as you wade through the plethora of choices. Many 'weight loss' supplements have not, from my experience, consistently confirmed their value. And when it comes to research, much of it is inconclusive or poorly performed or had results only when the participants were eating a highly restricted diet or they have only been tested in tubes or on lab animals. Mice and rats make good test subjects because their physiological response to disease and treatments is similar to humans. However, we are far more complex beings with larger brains and a multifarious relationship with food. Results on mice is not conclusive to humans until its been confirmed with solid research using people as subjects.

Having laid out my reservations to weight loss supplements, I also want to offer some hope, as there is some to be gleaned. Below, I offer you the best of the bunch, choosing to share with you only the products that meet a number of parameters: they have been tested on humans using randomized, placebo controlled, double-blind studies, the gold standard for research. They needed to show successful results without extreme calorie restriction – nothing under 1800 calories. They also need to be both safe, and have other benefits for your health. I focus on the ones that are the most likely to show you some results, and I caution you about all others that you may see on the internet or on TV. In most cases they won't be harmful but they will put a larger hole in your pocket. This includes hoodia, raspberry ketones, 7-keto, forskolin, guarana, L-carnitine, chitosan, and pyruvate. I am not saying that they absolutely won't work. I am just letting you know that at this time, in the fall of 2012, there are no randomized, double-blind, placebo controlled human trials that show conclusively that they do. One more word of caution; even the best supplements that I mention below will not provide you with lasting change over time if you do not do the other work to change your lifestyle. Homeostasis is a process of the body equalizing itself through feedback and regulation. Homeostasis will eventually drive your body to return to what it sees as a norm, thus a product that has good results initially will eventually lose its effect. If you don't prepare yourself with a foundation of good nutrition and an intimate understanding of your body, a magic pill will not get to your long-term goals. Life doesn't work that way. What is worth having doesn't come without working for it.

How you can do it

(I am offering you the following information for educational purposes only. You assume all responsibility for any outcome of choosing to follow one or more of the suggestions offered here. It would be best to consult with your practitioner before embarking on any supplement plan.)

Weight loss supplements can generally be divided into four primary actions.

1. Increasing your sense of satiation and suppressing your appetite, thus reducing cravings

2. Increasing metabolism and your body's ability to burn energy

3. Body sculpting

4. Starch absorption

Often they will have crossovers. Those that increase your metabolism will also reduce your appetite or cut cravings. Here are the best of the best.

Increasing Satiation and Suppressing Appetite

Eating frequently in the day, including fibre, particularly soluble fibre at each meal will go a long way to regulating your appetite and cravings. If you are however, fibre-challenged and you could use some help in this area, then here is my gold recommendation:

PGX

PGX is one of the most effective supplements that I know of, and has to date, seven human studies supporting its use for weight reduction, cholesterol lowering, stabilization of blood sugar and an increase in satiation hormones. This is one supplement that I do recommend on a regular basis, specifically for those who are having blood sugar symptoms and difficulty controlling their portion sizes and cravings. It can also be helpful to take it at night, before bed, to stabilize your blood sugar throughout the night, potentially improving your sleep. It is safe but should not be ingested at the same time of day that you take medications as it might block their effectiveness. Also as a soluble fibre, it can cause some digestive discomfort as your system is adjusting. Gas and bloating are not uncommon. I have found two ways to minimize this. One is to start slower, increasing your dose slowly over a two to three week period. The second is to take it on an empty stomach at least 30 minutes before meals, unlike the suggestion on the label.

- Forms: Capsules, or in powder form, or in combination with whey protein.
- Dosage: 2.5 – 5.0 grams, 3X/day on an empty stomach before meals, but always start with a low dose and increase as the gastrointestinal tract adjusts to the increase in fibre.

Increasing Metabolism and the Body's Capacity to Burn Energy

This is my favourite category because I find that the products that provide an increase in metabolism have the most beneficial effects. Plus these products tend to support a reduction in cravings as well. As with all supplements, start slowly and build up over one to two weeks to the recommended dose, allowing your body to adjust so that you can minimize any transient side effects.

Microfiltration Whey Isolate Powder

The first order of business in week one of *Jump Off the Diet Treadmill* was to eat more protein. I suggested protein shakes, including whey protein as the main source. Whey is actually a functional food disguised as a supplement. I want to go into more detail about it here so that you understand its value, why I recommend it to all of my clients (as long as they're not vegans or have a sensitivity to whey), and what you can look for if you decide to make use of it.

Do you remember the nursery rhyme "Little Miss Muffet sat on her tuffet eating her curds and whey..."? The curds and whey is a reference to the two proteins in milk, casein (curds) and whey. Cheese processing transforms the casein into curds. The by-product of this process is the whey. Whey is then processed, preferably by filtration to produce a highly concentrated protein source. Whey has been widely researched for its positive effects on bone, muscle, blood, brain, pancreas, immune, cancer, infection, metabolism, wound healing, learning, and aging. An entire book could be devoted to the benefits to be had from this substance, but we'll focus just on its effects related to weight.

Recall that protein stimulates the hormone glucagon, which stabilizes blood sugar in between meals and releases the sugar-fat molecule from the fat cells to be burned for fuel. Whey offers a super quick source of protein that is portable and highly bioavailable. In other words, our bodies find it easy to digest and make use of the protein fractions that are contained within it. One of these protein molecules is alpha lactalbumin. It is rich in tryptophan, which will stimulate serotonin production. You may recall that serotonin is the hormone that regulates our sleep, mood and appetite. If you have enough of it, cravings decrease, you feel happier and you sleep better. In fact, not only will you sleep better, but also you may wake up with greater alertness and capacity to concentrate. There is another protein molecule in whey called glycomacropeptide (GMP). Research demonstrates that whey protein, especially one that is rich in GMP improves satiation. GMP is touted to raise levels of CCK, one of our satiation hormones. CCK is also a crucial factor for digestion. It stimulates the pancreas to secrete digestive enzymes.

There are a lot of whey protein powders out there. You want to look for an isolate that has a higher concentration of protein and more purity than a concentrate. Also avoid ones that are processed via ion exchange. In this case, they will be prepared with heat or chemicals that will increase the sodium content and destroy some of the health promoting protein molecules, such as GMP and immune stimulating lactoferrin. Look on the ingredient list to ensure that it says that it is processed via cross-flow microfiltration or ultra cross-flow microfiltration. This method produces an undenatured whey that still contains GMP's and important immune enhancing nutrients. Watch out for any additional ingredients that are artificial, such as sweeteners and artificial flavourings.

+ Forms: powders

+ Dosage: 1 scoop of cross flow microfiltration whey isolate should provide between 25 – 35 g of protein, depending on the scoop that they provide in the container.

Green Tea Extract

There has been an abundance of research on green tea and its benefits as an antioxidant and anti-inflammatory, improving outcomes related to heart disease and arthritis. It is immune enhancing as a defense against bacteria and viruses, as well as a support against cancer. With all that green tea has going for it, it is worth noting its beneficial effects on fat loss as well. The research on humans has been solid, with many studies showing a significant lowering of total body fat mass, waist circumference, BMI, and insulin sensitivity within eight to twelve weeks. The major component having an effect on fat metabolism seems to be the catechins, particularly epigallocatechin gallate, thankfully shortened to EGCG.

Green tea in beverage form and the capsules of the extract, have both shown favourable results. However, there is an advantage to drinking the tea itself, in that it seems to show potential health benefits that the capsules don't, such as lowering LDL cholesterol. If you choose to drink the tea, you will need to aim for four cups (for a total of 32 ounces) per day to reach the amounts used in research. Less than that will still be helpful but the more you get, the more the catechins can do their work oxidizing your fat.

The quality of the tea also matters. Shabnam Weber, owner of 'The Tea Emporium' (www.theteaemporium.com) informed me that some teas have more catechins than others. Gyokuro, from Japan and Lung Ching Dragonwell, from China, are two green teas that have a higher ratio of buds plus the first two leaves that are closest to the buds, where the catechins are more abundant. If you are serious about using green tea as a catalyst to support your fat loss, then those options, if you can access them, would be a great choice. However any good quality green tea, or white for that matter, will be valuable. Note that most tea bags use the dregs of the leaves and will have far less bioactive components. Loose-leaf teas with larger pieces of leaf will have more medicinal qualities. If drinking that much tea is not feasible for you, then a capsule containing a variety of catechins with 20% EGCG is advisable. There are no known side effects but there is a fat loss advantage when used in conjunction with a dosage of caffeine.

- Forms: tea beverage, capsules
- Dosage: 4 cups of high quality green tea or 690 mg. of green tea catechins (35% ECGC) per day
  (Note that dosages of catechins and EGCG has been varied in successful studies. This dose offers an effective average.)

Green coffee bean extract
Although this supplement has only a small number of randomized placebo controlled studies to date, the results of one, in particular, are so impressive (despite it being a small sample) that it is worthy of mention. The subjects for this study were eight men and eight women, aged 22 – 46, with an average BMI of 28. This puts them in the overweight but not obese category. They were tested over a 22-week period with three arms of the study, in which they rotated taking either a high dose of 1050 mg per day, a low dose of 700 mg per day or a placebo. By the end of the 22 weeks, all subjects had taken the high dose, low dose and placebo for six weeks each, with a two-week 'washout' period in between. Despite making no changes to their lifestyle other than taking the supplement, all 16 subjects lost weight with 10 of the 16 losing a minimum of 10% of their body weight. Five lost at least 5% and one lost 4%. The green coffee bean used in the study was standardized for 45.9% chlorogenic acid, which influences glucose and fat metabolism. It is also what makes the green coffee bean unique compared to roasted coffee. The roasting of coffee beans destroys this valuable element, so although caffeine is associated with improvements in metabolism, it alone will not have the quality benefit that the green beans and chlorogenic acid have.

Like all the other supplements, start at a lower dose and increase slowly, while you observe its effects on your body. You might notice an increase in blood flow to your face or scalp or some jitteriness due to its stimulating effect.

- Forms: Capsules
- Dosage: 350 – 800 mg, 2X per day in between or before meals. If you are feeling the stimulating effects and are not comfortable with it, take them mid-meal.

Garcinia Cambogia

Garcinia is a fruit from southern India that contains an extract called hydroxycitric acid, HCA. In essence, HCA prevents the conversion of carbohydrate into fat by inhibiting an enzyme called ATP-citrate lyase. Garcinia may also turn on heat producing mechanisms to increase the breakdown of stored fat as well as suppress appetite through the release of serotonin. Some of the successful research on humans have been small trials and not randomized placebo controlled. However one study on 60 men and women over eight weeks on a 2000 calorie diet with a minimum of 30 minutes of walking, five times per week, reduced body weight by 5.4% and BMI by 5.2%, as well as improving other health parameters. The absorbability of the HCA might be the determining factor for its effectiveness. Normally HCA is bound to calcium, which on its own will inhibit its availability. However another form marketed as HCA-SX or Super CitriMax is balanced with a calcium-potassium mix that makes it entirely water-soluble and far more bioavailable. Research that generated positive results used that particular form, so if you are going to try it, I would suggest that you look for the product to contain the Super CitriMax form of HCA. It is likely that the outcome with Garcinia will be enhanced when taken with other ingredients such as green tea extract or green coffee bean.

- Forms: Capsules
- Dosage: 1555 mg of Garcinia cambogia, providing 933 mg. of HCA-SX, taken 3X per day, 30 – 60 minutes before meals daily, either alone or in a combination formula.

Body Sculpting

CLA (Conjugated Linoleic Acid)

CLA is a type of Omega-6 fat that is normally present in beef and dairy that have been pastured-raised. The CLA itself depends on the grass, in order to be formed in the fat of the animal. It is also found in eggs and strangely enough, the only non-animal food -- select mushrooms, such as the common button mushroom. In supplement form it is most commonly derived from safflower oil. The actions of CLA are not entirely known, although it is thought to block an enzyme, lipoprotein lipase that stores dietary fat in your fat cells while it activates a different enzyme which enhances metabolism of fat in the muscles. Research on CLA has mostly resulted in the reduction of body fat in the abdomen although some research showed a bigger change in women and more loss in the thighs. CLA seems to exert greater effects on those who are obese, with a BMI of 30 plus. In the past there has been some concern for the safety of CLA use. Since then, however, there have been two trials, one for six and another for twelve months. They confirmed the safety of CLA, although there was a slight rise in LDL cholesterol in the one year study. This may be due to the increase in the Omega-6 to Omega-3 ratio and specifically a shift in the DHA levels in the heart tissue. My suggestion would be to increase your intake of fish oil along with the consumption of CLA and limit your use to six months. Abdominal side effects, if you get them, will likely lessen with use.

+ Form: Capsules
+ Dosage: 3400 – 3600 mg. per day, taken in divided dosages with food.

Starch Blocking

Phaseolamin

Phaseolamin is an extract of the common white bean (Phaseolus vulgaris) that is sold on the market as Phase 2. It is able to reduce spikes in blood sugar after eating a carb rich meal by inhibiting an enzyme, alpha-amylase that helps to break down carbohydrates. At least ten clinical studies have demonstrated weight loss with Phase 2, some of those proving to be quite significant. As an example, in a study with 60 participants, the subjects averaged a 10.5% reduction in body fat after only 30 days, even though they were eating a carbohydrate rich 2000 – 2200 calorie diet. This supplement is particularly good for those who have their starchy and sweet comfort foods that they can't seem to get a handle on. It is also a good option for overindulgent events and holidays. Like some of the other supplements, it has an adjustment period. It is not unusual to have bloating and gas in the first weeks of using it. Start slowly, taking only one 500 mg. dose before meals. You can increase to take one before each carb rich meal and then as much as two per meal. This is not an excuse to go wild on carbs, but it will take the pressure off for those special treats. Think of it as a backup during particularly challenging times, rather than a constant.

+ Forms: Capsules, chewables, powder

- Dosage: Take 500 – 3000 mg. per day (use divided dosages as you get into higher amounts). Take before or right after meals.

One final word of caution regarding weight loss supplements: I have noticed that people can get so hopeful about the benefits of what they're taking that they give themselves A LOT more room to indulge. This will not work. Think of a supplement as an adjunct to healthy eating and living. It may support your good efforts but it will not substitute for them.

Set Up Your Environment
for Long-term Success

What you need to do

Lasting change doesn't happen without shifts in both our internal and external environment. Throughout this book, hints for changing your surroundings have been peppered in with the internal shifts in how you eat, think, feel and move. Often those changes have been small adjustments that make it easier to take action. Putting a pitcher of water and glass on your desk to remind you to drink, making arrangements to workout with a buddy, using a smaller plate for better portion control. These are simple actions. KISS, 'keep it simple, sweetie' is profoundly unsophisticated, and usable. It is easier to transform your habits for the better by altering your environment in small ways.

Imagine yourself taking three weeks to go to a luxury spa that specializes in detox and weight loss. While there, your healthy meals are prepared for you under the supervision of a chef and nutritionist. You go to exercise class and yoga every day. You spend time walking in the surrounding hills. You luxuriate in the water spas and steam room and follow that with a massage. There is time to read and nap. You also attend classes to learn about nutrition, healthy cooking, detoxification, and behavioral change. Everyone around you is doing the same program, cells phones are prohibited in public spaces, internet time is limited to one hour per day and there is no TV.

How much easier would it be to lose weight and maintain it if you spent all your time in that environment? Kind of a no-brainer, isn't it. Easier, yes, but for just about all of us, that is not our reality. The point to be made is that in the right environment, your choices would be clearer.

To that end, this week is about a focused observation of your environment to see what stands in the way of you reaching your goals and sustaining them. Consider how you can switch those obstacles from impenetrable brick walls to ones that now have a doorway (even if the knob does get stuck sometimes) that you can walk through. Where change is needed, you'll need to look at what's working for you and what might be missing.

When you are looking to redesign some aspect of your life, it is the small shifts that are made in both your internal and external environment, that over time, lead to big change.

Why you need to do this

When I was looking at the research to support this section of the book, I was surprised by what I found. I had assumed that people are influenced by the behaviours of others in their environment. But what appears more conclusive is that us humans are motivated by what is considered normal for our environment. This is an important distinction when you're thinking about your surrounding influences and how you can change the norm.

In 2007, Nicholas Christakis, M.D., Ph.D., M.P.H., and James H. Fowler, Ph.D. published a study in The New England Journal of Medicine citing the results of their investigation of 12,067 people over a thirty-two year period from 1971 to 2003. They wanted to observe whether obesity would spread over social networks. What they found was enlightening. Amongst mutual friends, if one friend became obese, the likelihood of the other, also becoming obese increased by 171%. If a sibling of the same sex became obese, the risk for sisters increased by 67% and for brothers by 44%. Amongst married couples it was an increase of 37%. What was most astonishing, however, is that in all cases, geography was not a deciding factor. The risk was there whether they were in close proximity to each other or not. What this means is that it wasn't a continuous imitation of behavior that made the difference. Rather, as the researchers point out, it suggests that the spread of obesity may rely more on a change in what is considered an acceptable norm.

This may account then, at least in part, for the epidemic in overweight and obesity worldwide. We may not consider it desirable to be fat. Yet the reality is that two out of three people in the US and almost the same ratio in Canada and the UK are overweight, which makes someone who is heavy, part of the crowd rather than an outsider. It is far more acceptable to be fat now than it was in the 60's, 70's or 80's, because it is now the norm. Human beings need to feel like they belong.

Fashion trends exemplify how what is considered normal, ultimately drives behaviour. The teenage boy who wears his pants below his butt with his underwear exposed does not do it because he watched his peers get dressed that morning, but because he has seen it enough times to know that it is the norm for 'cool' guys (or what he perceives as cool for his social circle).

Our desire to belong and be seen as normal is woven into our genetics and our survival. In days past, when we depended (in more obvious ways) on our community for our food and sustenance, being ostracized from our pack meant probable starvation and threat by the elements and wild beast. Although our stressors are different today, you might be able to get a feel for our ingrained wiring by imagining what you would encounter if you were to wear attire to work that was absolutely outside of the norm. Envision, as a man, dressing in the garb of an Englishman from the early 18th century. You would sport breeches to your knees, stockings to meet them, a long waistcoat, white frilly lace shirt, and don't forget, a curly white wig. As a woman, you would wear a tight bodice and petticoat and your hair would be pinned up in an elaborate 'do.' You would, without a doubt, stand out in the crowd. There would be stares, sneers and inquiries. At best, most would just find it funny. At worst, depending on your community, someone may want to beat you up.

Any movement far away from the norm will take us outside of our comfort zone. Too far out and we're not going to do it. Therefore, when considering change, you want to make things simple and easily accessible by altering your surroundings in ways that don't cause too much stress. This is where the 'keep it simple, sweetie' comes in.

Whether we're adjusting to the norm or considering the behaviours behind it, clearly us human beings are social creatures who are powerfully influenced by our environment and those who are in it. Habits, good and bad, will proliferate depending on the conduct that is deemed acceptable and preferable by our social circles. If your workplace has done an about-face to create a healthier work environment by changing the lunch options in the cafeteria to salads and grilled chicken rather than burgers and fries, a new norm will be created that will make it easier to make good choices. Joining a morning walking group, a mothers and babies fitness class, making a family decision that three meals per week will be eaten together around the dinner table, rather than in front of the television, are all shifts in the environment that will support sustainable goals.

How you can do it

Lucy is a young woman in her twenties who attended one of my group programs. At the beginning of our eight weeks together, she shared with us that one of her biggest challenges was hanging out with her friends when their social life centered around going out for food and drinks. In brainstorming her options, she agreed to talk with them to see if they could support her. Not only did her friends agree but they took it on as an opportunity for adventure. Over the eight weeks that our group met, they had shifted from going out to eat three times a week to taking turns coming up with new experiences that they could have. They explored different parts of the city on foot, played ping pong at a trendy Spin club, went to speed dating evenings, bowled, went dancing and met at art openings. Sometimes, they followed their

adventures by going to a restaurant, but they chose ones
that had healthy options and spent less time there so that
the consumption was minimized. Lucy was thrilled that her
friends had taken up the request with such gusto. She said
that it not only helped her reach her weight loss goal, it also
shifted the fun quotient for their social life.

Needless to say, most of us will have more challenges to deal with than Lucy did. It is worth noting however, that Lucy was willing to take the risk to ask for support to create the conditions that would promote her success.

Sometimes you will have to be the change-maker, the initiator. Other times you will need to find situations where you can follow others. In either case, it is about surrounding yourself with an environment in which you can relax, so that your need for self-control doesn't have to be on constant alert. You can start by choosing options that are easy to do, that will minimize the stress of creating change. Think of the 'low hanging fruit' – the fruit that is easiest to pick. Go for that. If getting more exercise is a challenge for you, choosing to take the stairs in your building at work may be the starting point. If you're on the 36th floor, then get off at the 26th or the 30th or whatever you feel you can handle. If drinking enough water has always eluded you, then add in one extra glass first thing in the morning as a start. Create more environmental support by having your glass out on the counter so it is the first thing you notice in the morning. Small changes make a big difference and over time will lead to new habits.

Plan for your environment. Set it up with specific intentions. In the book, *Switch: How to Change Things When Change is Hard*, authors Chip and Dan Heath talk about the research of psychologist, Peter Gollwitzer. He refers to 'preloading a decision.' Preloading sets up a trigger that will make it easier to follow through on actions that you know you need to do. You could also call it intention setting, or 'when/then' planning. *When* I arrive at work, *then* I will walk the stairs. *When* we finish dinner, *then* we will go for a walk. *When* my reminder alarm goes off at 11:30, *then* I'll leave for the noon bootcamp class. Gollwitzer says that, "when people pre-decide, they pass the control of their behaviour on to the environment. Action triggers protect goals from tempting distractions, bad habits, or competing goals." When you set an intention, that intention becomes part of your environment.

As you set up your self-care action triggers, keep in mind that they will be more powerful when they are specific, rather than general. In the training to become a life coach, that concept was drilled into us. People need to be specific if they are going to be successful at following through. 'Keep it simple, sweetie' reflects our brain's need for a clear neural pathway. As an example, saying, "I'm going to walk to and from work everyday this week, rain or shine," is clearer than, "I'm going to walk five times this week." Deciding that, "I'm going to drink only two, five ounce glasses of wine throughout the entire night," is more powerful than, "I'm going to cut down on my wine tonight."

As you explore the different layers of your environment below, consider which ones you can most easily tame. What are some initial steps that would have an immediate impact, even if it's small? One of the mistakes that people often make when it comes to their environment is that they think that if they can't change the most challenging aspects immediately, then they can't succeed. I have had conversations with many people who have expressed an interest in losing weight who also say that they can't do it because their husband or wife is resistant. If that's the case, don't start with your partner. If you are serious about making change, think small steps. What can you take charge of right now? Then when you have that figured out, what can you do next? As much as we can all sympathize with the challenge, if you blame your husband, wife or work environment for your own behaviours, you will remain a victim of your circumstance instead of being the initiator of change. You may have to be the one to create a new norm. But as you blaze a new trail, don't start climbing at the steepest part of the path. Instead start from the flats where you can breath easier.

I worked with a young professional woman a number of years back. In her initial session, she said that her husband was a huge challenge for her. He was a meat and potatoes kind of guy who was not open-minded and hated vegetables. They also tended to spend a lot of time in front of the

TV together. Since their marriage three years previously, she had gained forty pounds. She wasn't keen on cooking two meals every night (after she came home from her full-time work) so she decided to start with the places that she had more control. She walked to work, prepared or bought healthy lunches for herself, and went to the gym two times a week. When she was home alone, she turned off the TV and did some journaling, read or spent time on the computer doing things that she enjoyed. When her husband was there, she continued to eat with him and hang out watching TV. But after a few months of this, with some good changes under her belt, she wanted to go to the next level. She got stronger about her own needs and told him that she wouldn't continue making meat and potatoes every night, that she wanted variety. He started eating out more and she was socializing with friends more frequently. It was clear that she was getting stronger and more independent. Eight months after she started working with me, they decided to get a divorce. Her evolvement would naturally have an effect on her environment. But she couldn't have started with the biggest challenge, which was getting out of an unhappy marriage. She had to begin with what she felt ready for.

Not everyone who has a resistant partner ends up divorcing them. More often than not there is a happy ending. The positive influence of one person has a beneficial impact on the people around them. It's understandable, because when they witness the higher energy levels, better state of mind, and loss of weight that happens in the person they love, they are inspired to make changes themselves. For this reason, whenever you can, engage your family, friends, and colleagues in your goals. Ask them for help. Fearlessly spread the new norm and the behaviours that go along with it. Good habits are as contagious as bad ones.

Now let's consider where you can start with your environment and what influences are in it.

Imagine for a moment that you are standing by the side of a pond, where the water is clear and still as glass. You drop a stone into the pond and watch the waves ripple outwards in concentric circles, dissipating as they get further from the center.

We can use this metaphor of the stone and circles to identify your environment. You are the stone at the center of pond. Each ripple outwards creates a circle that surrounds you. The closer that circle is to the center (you) the stronger its influence on you and you on it. As it ripples further outward, the influence dissipates, but it's present nonetheless.

The circles of influence regarding our self-care, from the center outwards, are most commonly in this order:

- **Family and home** – this is whomever you live with as well as other family members that you are connected to, whether it is your parents, siblings, grandparents, or another, whether you live with them or not. It also includes your home environment, what foods are there, what activities you do -- on your own or with someone else.

- **Friends and leisure** – these are the people, both male and female, that you hang out with, speak to, share your life with outside of your family. If you have a boyfriend or girlfriend that you don't live with, they are in this circle. This includes the leisure activities that you do with your friends.

- **Colleagues and work** – consider your work space, who you share it with, who you report to, management, owners, the general work environment, access to food, support systems for your health, work hours, expectations.

- **Community and activities** – outside of your immediate family and friends, do you have a group that you're involved with? It could be others that you are affiliated with re: health, charities, religion, game playing, etc. This is the physical environment, the attitudes and the food that you share with these groups.

⬥ **Media and information** – this is all of the sources that you get your knowledge from re: health and other aspects of life and news that might affect your health: internet, radio, television, books, courses, etc. The affect of this circle may be more insidious or beneficial in ways that may not be as obvious. However note the impact they have on you. Do they provide effective support or do they overwhelm you?

Note that in the research by Christakis and Fowler that I mentioned previously, they identified that mutual friends of the same sex and siblings of the same sex had a greater influence on the risk of sharing obesity than a mate does. This may be the case for you as well. The two inner circles then, are interchangeable and will depend on the person. In fact, you may have a different order regarding all of your circles of influence. You need to identify that for yourself. The order is less relevant than the recognition of the different aspects of your environment that play a role in your choices.

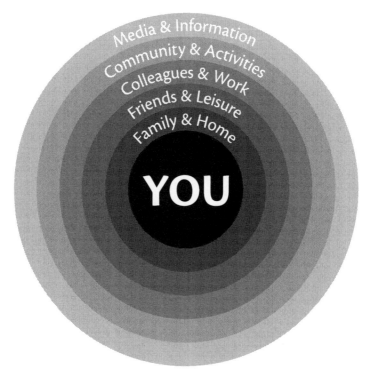

Think about each circle of influence in your environment in relation to your health and weight loss goals.

* What assets exist in each circle that work to support the goals that you have?

* What obstacles are getting in your way?

* What can you do, at this point, to make those obstacles less intrusive?

* What might be missing that would help you out?

Some examples might be helpful:

* *

* *Aisha has two sons and a husband at home. She recognized that one of the obstacles in her environment that was causing her some challenge was the junk food that she buys for her kids. When bags of chips and pretzels are around and everyone else is eating them, she is inclined to join in. Fortunately for her, one of her assets in her home environment is the support of her family. So she decided to get them on board to help her. She told them her dilemma and together they decided that first of all, they wouldn't have as much junk food (although they didn't want to give it up all together). Secondly, that when they did have it while watching TV, they would make her popcorn so that she could munch on something that was less of an issue for her. Also, when she felt the temptation of the chips, they would tease her and remind her of her goals. She reported that they did all this with great humor. What a great asset!!*

* *One of Ken's obstacles was getting enough exercise in the midst of a seventy-hour work week. He also missed having a*

social life outside of his clients and workplace. He had lost touch with a circle of friends that were avid cross-country cyclists. To get back in shape, he decided to tap into that asset. He made arrangements to go out with them on their next ride. He labored to keep up, but he didn't mind. It felt great to be back on the bike again after years of being caught in his lawyer work. He now prioritizes rides with them two to three times per week.

- *Michelle lives out in the country but she comes into the city twice per week to work with clients. On those days, she was spending so much of her extra time in the car that her obstacle was her schedule. There just wasn't time to make it to a gym or to travel anywhere else to get exercise. That was until she mentioned the issue in passing to one of the men at the firm she works with. He uses the stairs, twenty-five flights worth, to train for the mountain climbing and marathons that he does in better weather. They made a deal that they would do them together. She is fine with being many flights behind him. She just loves the feeling of working her heart, breathing hard, and appreciates the accountability that he offers.*

- *Marcia commutes into downtown from an outlying suburb. She spends one hour on the train each way. She turned this into an asset. She decided that instead of playing on her mobile phone she would take the time to meditate or listen to inspirational books or visualizations. It relieves her stress and gives her the energy she needs to better deal with a less than harmonious family life.*

- *With three young kids, Meg couldn't prioritize the finances to join a gym. She also felt guilty if she took too much time away from her children's lives to get exercise. She had a close friend who had a similar situation so together they created an asset. They started a meet-up group in their suburban neighborhood that was focused on 'Mom's After-Kids-in-Bed Bootie Camp'. A community rec center agreed to let them use a room in the basement for free. They also hired a trainer who was just starting out and agreed to do a one-hour class for next to nothing, just for the opportunity to get more experience. They meet twice per week and have a great time while getting an evening workout.*

Sometimes you'll need to get creative within your environment. Ask yourself, is there someone you can follow? Or do you need to initiate the change?

Either way, go for it. What do you have to lose? Other than a wee bit o' weight.

Addendum

- - - - - - - - - - - - - -

10 Physical Issues that will Stop You from Losing Weight (Despite Your Best Efforts)

- - -

Further Reading

- - -

Resources and End Notes

10 Physical Issues that will Stop You from Losing Weight (Despite Your Best Efforts)

Nutrition, exercise, sleep, energy management, thoughts and emotions all contribute to how well someone can lose weight and keep it off. Sometimes however, despite a person's best efforts in these areas, something still blocks the loss of fat. This section reviews the physiological issues that can be at the heart of stubborn weight loss. Keep in mind that these disturbances rarely happen alone. More commonly you find one or more of these present at the same time.

Also note that if any of these issues apply to you, all of what has been presented in this book will be a crucial part of your healing. You won't go wrong by following this program. However, with therapeutic issues, the support of one or more skilled practitioners may be a key to full recovery.

1. Blood Sugar Imbalance

I mentioned this numerous times in the program, particularly in the weeks devoted to protein, breakfast, and carbohydrates. Fat is one of the body's fuel sources, along with proteins and carbohydrate. The hormones insulin and glucagon play a sensitive dance in the storage of glucose (blood sugar) as fat and its release so that it can be burned as energy. Too much insulin release or an insensitivity of the cells to be receptive to insulin, will upset that balance and keep fat tightly tucked away. If you are dealing with any form of blood sugar dysregulation, including diabetes, PCOS, metabolic syndrome, insulin resistance, hypo or hyperglycemia, it would serve you well to get some added support.

2. Sluggish Thyroid

The thyroid gland is like a thermometer regulating thermogenesis (heat production) and cellular metabolism. If the thyroid is sluggish, every cell in the body will be operating at a diminished capacity. Your body's calorie burning capacity will be reduced, leading to weight gain and fat storage. Unfortunately the standard blood test for thyroid function, the measure of thyroid stimulating hormone, TSH, does not tell the whole story of what's going on with this gland and its multiple hormones. Symptoms such as low body temperature, cold hands and feet, high cholesterol, low energy, feeling worse after exercise, and a thinning of the eyebrows from the outside edge are just a few of the indicators that there may be something going on with this important metabolic gland.

3. Adrenal Insufficiency

The adrenal glands help us adapt to stress, and are directly affected by chronic stress. Cortisol, one of the powerful hormones released by the adrenals, stimulates the breakdown of protein from our tissues, thus reducing our calorie burning capacity. It also triggers the fat-storage enzymes telling them to keep that fat right where we don't want it. Cortisol fuels the hunger signals in our brain which trigger us to overeat. It is possible to have too much or too little cortisol activity. Either way, you could be plagued with anxiety, fatigue, the challenge of getting up in the morning, insomnia, belly fat, immune issues and a host of other complaints. With our high stress lifestyles, adrenal insufficiency is a common issue.

4. Yeast Infections and/or Parasites

If the terrain of our gastrointestinal tract is lacking its normal immune defenses, then our body becomes susceptible to overgrowth of yeast and/ or parasitic invasion. This can be a major (and often unknown) reason for increased appetite, intense sugar, carbs and alcohol cravings, weight gain, low energy and a general lack of well-being. There will commonly be digestive discomfort such as gas, constipation or loose stools, bloating, and cramping. Toenail and skin fungus, vaginal yeast infections, itchy ears and eyes, foggy head, and sore throats are often present as well. If organisms are on board, they need to be dealt with before sustainable weight loss and optimal health can be reached.

5. Food Intolerances

Wheat and other gluten grains, yeast, sugar, dairy, soy, eggs, citrus, chocolate and corn are examples of common food allergens. Eating a food that you are intolerant to, can slow down metabolism, cause bloating or other digestive disturbances and raise insulin levels, all contributors to fat storage. Symptoms are commonly digestive ones, similar to those mentioned above under yeast/parasites. The respiratory system is often weakened as well so that you'll experience airborne allergies, chronic throat clearing or coughs, sinus congestion and frequent colds and flus.

6. Toxic Overload

If the eliminative organs; the liver, lymph, kidneys and colon are congested, the toxins that are not being sent out as waste are commonly stored in the fat cells, wrecking havoc on cellular metabolism and inhibiting fat loss. Any number of symptoms can show up: headaches, body odor, bad breath, intolerance to fatty foods are just a few of the possibilities. Improper elimination may show itself in your skin via acne, eczema, hives or other eruptions.

7. Depleted Brain Chemistry

I have frequently mentioned brain chemistry, particularly the neurotransmitters, dopamine, serotonin and GABA. Lacking a balance in one or more of these leads to mood swings, anxiety, apathy and depression as well as more serious mental illness. Depleted neurochemicals are a physiological link to emotional eating and food cravings.

8. Hormone Imbalance

Hormones are released by the endocrine glands, travel through the blood, and act as the chemical messengers as they find their way to target organs and tissues. They interrelate in a network, so even a small deviation in normal function of any hormone can result in system-wide changes in energy production, stress responses and weight gain or retention. Particularly crucial are the reproductive steroid hormones, testosterone, progesterone and estrogen. Symptoms include PMS, hot flashes, decreased sex drive and function, a loss of muscle mass, insomnia plus others.

9. Enzyme, Vitamin and Mineral Deficiencies

Enzymes are needed for every metabolic function of the body, including digestion. When food is not being broken down properly with the help of enzymes, it causes a chain reaction of digestive dysfunction. This can result in more stress to the linings of the gastrointestinal tract, eliminative organs, particularly the liver and colon, an imbalance in the intestinal flora, and a lack of optimal system functions throughout the body. Along with the enzymes, the vitamins and minerals are co-factors in the workings of every body system, including energy production and metabolism of protein, carbs and fat. There are so many possible symptoms associated with nutrient deficiencies, too many to mention. However, with an analysis of your blood chemistry, looking at optimal ranges, in conjunction with a thorough overview of your symptoms, it is possible to determine your ideal diet and therapeutic needs.

10. Fatty Acid Deficiency

As you may have garnered by now, there are good fats and bad fats. The essential fatty acids, Omega 3 and Omega 6, are the good fats that we must get from our diet and are crucial to metabolism. The formation and function of the hormones, all cell membranes, including brain cells, protection of internal organs, the luster of hair and skin, and fertility all require the good fats. If you want to maintain energy, mental stability, sex drive, muscle strength, bowel regularity, and avoid carbohydrate cravings, you need an ample supply of good fats. If you're getting an adequate supply and you still seem to suffer from symptoms of fat deficiency, your digestive capacity to break down and absorb the fats may be compromised.

A Final Note

If you have any symptoms that are of concern, you will do well to start with the processes in Jump Off the Diet Treadmill. You can begin anywhere that speaks to you, taking on what you feel you can handle. Then one step at a time, continue to modify. If at any point, you feel stuck and need guidance, my suggestion is to seek out an expert for support.

Be fearless in your search for optimal wellness. You'll be rewarded with a healthy relationship with food and a strong body.

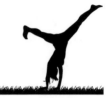

Further Reading

Jump Off the Treadmill includes so many aspects of whole health that I can only touch the surface of many of them. For some topics, you will find enough to get you going and it may be all that you need for now. For others, it is probable that some of you may want to delve more deeply with the help of other teachers and experts in their field. To that end, and in honor of some of the coaches, doctors, therapists, healers and researchers who have been a teacher and an inspiration to me, I am including a few favorite resources below. They are in no particular order.

The Diet Cure by Julia Ross

I find the title of this book deceiving. You might surmise from it that it is about dieting. On the contrary. It does however focus on good nutrition as a central component to the healing of out- of-balance brain chemistry. Ross is a clinical psychologist who heads up a California-based clinic that specializes in addiction, eating and weight disorders using nutrient and biochemical therapy along with counseling and education. I think it is one of the best layperson books for understanding the physiology behind addiction.

Mind/Body Nutrition (CD set), The Slow Down Diet: Eating for Pleasure, Energy and Weight Loss or Nourishing Wisdom: A Mind-Body Approach to Nutrition and Well Being by Marc David

I love this guy. He has been an inspiration from afar. As a Nutritional Psychologist and the founder of The Institute for the Psychology of Eating (www.psychologyofeating.com), you can guess where his expertise and passion lay. If you are interested in furthering your understanding about the mind body connection and how it directly affects your relationship with food, then his work is a must-read.

Shrink Yourself: Break Free from Emotional Eating Forever by Roger Gould, M.D.

I am impressed with the thoroughness and simple language that Dr. Gould uses to help his readers understand the emotional patterns that keep them stuck on food. He also offers the tools to change those patterns. My approach is more body-based, not so analytical. I think there is room for and a need for both. Some people will respond to one more than the other. This is the best book that I have read on the analytical process related to emotional eating.

Anatomy of the Spirit: The Seven Stages of Power and Healing by Caroline Myss, Ph.D.

As a medical intuitive who has worked closely with physicians, Caroline Myss is one of the most well respected teachers of energetic medicine. In this book, she lays out how your mental, emotional and spiritual life are reflected in the chakras or energy organs of your body. She is grounded, logical and straightforward. Highly recommend it if you looking for a deeper understanding of health, healing and holism.

Switch: How to Change Things When Change is Hard by Chip Heath and Dan Heath

The Heath brothers are so good at metaphor, storytelling and clarifying processes that their book reads almost like fiction. A fascinating overview of how us human beings operate, and options for making it easier to help ourselves and others make changes, whether it's personal or in an organizational setting.

A User's Guide to the Brain by John Ratey, M.D.

If you are as fascinated by the brain as I am, then this is a great reference. It offers an overview of the anatomy and function of the brain in easy to understand language with enough stories to make it accessible.

Nutrition Almanac, 5th Edition by Lavon J. Dunne

I frequently use this book as a reference for the nutritional values of specific foods. It also has a section on healing imbalances and what foods to use to do that. My earmarked pages are the ones that lay out the nutrient composition of specific foods, organized within their food groups. It includes protein, carbohydrates, fibre, each of the vitamins, minerals, and the breakdown of the fat and amino acid profiles.

The 150 Healthiest Foods On Earth by Jonny Bowden, Ph.D., C.N.S.

This book is yummy. It is laid out with glossy pages and beautiful photos. Bowden creates books as good as the food he recommends. In this case, he combined his own review of what the top health foods are with a survey of many of his colleagues who are well-known experts in nutrition and health, asking them what they eat. The result is a fun and informative walk-though the world of natural foods. Makes a great gift.

Younger (Thinner) You Diet by Eric R. Braverman, MD

Dr. Braverman has written a number of books, all with a focus on brain health and nutritional therapy to support the brain. Here, he offers an interesting take on weight loss from the perspective of neurotransmitter deficiency. It may be clearer for you from reading this whether you need to focus on dopamine, serotonin, GABA or acetylcholine enhancement. It offers healing foods, spices and recipes for each.

The End of Overeating: Taking Control of the Insatiable North American Appetite by David A. Kessler, MD

A treatise on how the food industry markets, sells and gets us hooked on their foods. The fattening of our continent is a sad story but Kessler makes it readable and even light-hearted. His tone is curious, compassionate, and investigative. What results is an eye-opening view inside of our cravings and the industry that manipulates it.

Adrenal Fatigue: The 21st Century Stress Syndrome
by James L. Wilson, N.D., D.C., Ph.D

Adrenal issues may turn out to be the great epidemic of our modern era, walking side by side with obesity. Even though it is not widely recognized in standard medical practice, natural practitioners are addressing the issue head on. Dr. Wilson presents a through overview and makes this book shine with his full treatment of the healing process.

Precision Nutrition www.precisionnutrition.com
led by Dr. John Berardi

Berardi and his team are, from my experience, the most extensive source of information about nutrition on weight loss and fitness that can be found on the web. They offer a blend of science and coaching for behavioural change. They have a year-long group program for weight loss that is the envy of all solo coaches. Well, at least it is for me. They offer something that only a dedicated team can do.

Resources and Endnotes

Week 1 – Make Friends with Protein

* Grains and legumes/beans are each lacking one of the essential amino acids that make a complete protein. These essential amino acids are not manufactured in our body – we must get them from food. In the case of whole grains, it is most commonly the essential amino acid, lysine that is deficient. In beans it is another amino acid, methionine. Eaten together the grains and beans form a complete source of all of the essential amino acids. This is particularly crucial to understand if someone chooses to be vegan, thus eliminating all animal proteins from their diet. There is less need to focus on this issue if animal proteins are eaten daily, as they will provide all of the essential amino acids. Amaranth and buckwheat are the only two grains that provide a complete protein profile, including enough lysine. Quinoa provides an abundance of lysine but is lacking in two other essential amino acids, tryptophan and methionine, that can be made up by combining it with any of the other grains.

Berardi, John. *Precision Nutrition*, Toronto: Precision Nutrition Inc., 2000 – 2009.

King, Brad. *Fat Wars Action Planner.* Toronto: Wiley, 2003.

Te Morenga, L, and Mann, J. "The role of high-protein diets in body weight management and health." *The British Journal of Nutrition*, 2012 Aug;108 Suppl 2:S130-8.

Westerterp-Plantenga, MS, Lemmens, SG, and Westerterp, KR. "Dietary protein - its role in satiety, energetics, weight loss and health." *The British Journal of Nutrition*, 2012 Aug;108 Suppl 2:S105-12.

Wycherley, TP, Moran, LJ, Clifton, PM, Noakes, M, and Brinkworth, GD. "Effects of energy-restricted high-protein, low-fat compared with standard-protein, low-fat diets: a meta-analysis of randomized controlled trials." *American Journal of Clinical Nutrition*, 2012 Dec;96(6):1281-98.

Week 1 – Find Your Motivation

Brizendine, Louann. *The Female Brain*. Great Britain: Bantam Press, 2007.

Heath, Chip, and Health, Dan. *Switch: How to Change Things When Change is Hard*. New York: Random House, 2010.

Kaplan, F, Oudeyer, PV. "In Search of the Neural Circuits of Intrinsic Motivation." *Frontiers in Neuroscience*, 2007 November; 1(1): 225-236.

Ratey, John. *A User's Guide to the Brain: Perception, Attention, and the Four Theaters of the Brain*. New York: Vintage Books, 2002.

Rossman, Martin. "Imagery: Learning to Use the Mind's Eye." In *Mind, Body Medicine: How to Use your Mind for Better Health*. Edited by Goleman, Daniel and Gurin, Joel. Consumer Reports Books, 1993.

Ryan, Richard M., and Deci, Edward, L. "Intrinsic and Extrinsic Motivations: Classic Definitions and New Directions." *Contemporary Educational Psychology*, 2000; 25, 54 – 67.

Sample, Ian. "New year's resolutions doomed to failure, say psychologists." http://www.guardian.co.uk/lifeandstyle/2009/dec/28/new-years-resolutions-doomed-failure .

Week #2 – Eat Breakfast and Keep Eating

Howarth, NC, Saltzman, E, and Roberts, SB. "Dietary fibre and weight regulation." Nutrition Review, 2001 May; 59(5):129-39.

Koletzko, B, and Toschke, AM. "Meal patterns and frequencies: do they affect body weight in children and adolescents?" *Critical Reviews in Food Science and Nutrition*, 2010 February; 50 (2): 100-5.

McGuire, MT, Wing, RR, Klem, ML, and Hill, JO. "Behavioral strategies of individuals who have maintained long-term weight losses." *Obesity Research*, 1999 July;7(4):334-41.

National Weight Control Registry, Research findings available at http://www.nwcr.ws/Research/default.htm.

Week #2 – Be Accountable to Someone Other than Yourself

Gibbs, Jeanne. *Tribes: A new way of learning and being together.* Center Source Systems, LLC, 2001.

Hollis, JF, et al. "Weight Loss During the Intensive Intervention Phase of the Weight-Loss Maintenance Trial" *American Journal of Preventive Medicine*, 2008 August; 35 (2): 118 – 126.

Johnson, DW, and Johnson, R. *Cooperation and competition: Theory and research.* Interaction Book Company, 1989.

Kaiser Permanente Center for Health Research. "CHR Study Finds Keeping Food Diaries Doubles Weight Loss," 2008. Available at http://www.kpchr.org/research/public/News.aspx?NewsID=3.

Online experiment led by Professor Richard Wiseman, as reported at http://www.guardian.co.uk/science/2007/dec/28/sciencenews.research and http://www.guardian.co.uk/lifeandstyle/2009/dec/28/new-years-resolutions-doomed-failure

Week #3 – Commit to Upping Your Water Intake

* Adapted from www.watercure.com.

Batmanghelidj, F. *Your Body's Many Cries for Water: You're Not Sick, You're Thirsty. Don't Treat Thirst with Medication.* Falls Church, VA: Global Health Solutions, 1997.

Blum, JW, Jacobsen, DJ, and Donnelly, JE. "Beverage consumption patterns in elementary school aged children across a two-year period." *Journal of the American College of Nutrition*, 2005 Apr;24(2):93-8.

Fowler, Sharon, et.al, "Diet soda linked to weight gain in the elderly." *San Antonio Longitudinal Study of Aging*, 2011 American Diabetes Association (ADA) 71st Scientific Sessions: Abstract 0062-OR. Presented June 25, 2011.

Green, E, and Murphy, C. "Altered processing of sweet taste in the brain of diet soda drinkers." *Physiology & Behavior*, 2012 Nov 5;107(4):560-7.

Ingram, Colin. *The Drinking Water Book: A Complete Guide to Safe Drinking Water.* Berkeley, CA: Ten Speed Press, 1995.

Institute of Medicine. *Dietary reference intakes for water, potassium, sodium, chloride, and sulfate.* Washington, D.C.: The National Academies Press: 2004.

Week #3, Stop Beating Yourself Up

Baumeister, Roy, Bratslavsky, Ellen, Finkenauer, Catrin, and Vohs, Kathleen. "Bad is Stronger than Good." *Review of General Psychology*, 2001, Vol. 5, No. 4, 323 – 370.

Heath, Chip, and Health, Dan. *Switch: How to Change Things When Change is Hard.* New York: Random House, 2010.

Larsen, BA, et al. "The immediate and delayed cardiovascular benefits of forgiving." *Psychosomatic Medicine*, 2012 Sep;74(7):745-50.

Neff, K. D. "Development and validation of a scale to measure self-compassion." *Self and Identity*, 2003; 2, 223-250.

Worthington, EL, Witvliet, CV, Pietrini, P, and Miller, AJ. "Forgiveness, health, and well-being: a review of evidence for emotional versus decisional forgiveness, dispositional forgivingness, and reduced unforgiveness." *Journal of Behavioral Medicine*, 2007 Aug;30(4):291-302.

Week #4 – Eat close to Nature

* One might argue that 'we are what we absorb' and although I would agree with that, for the sake of this step in the program, we will be focusing on what you intake rather than concerning ourselves with how well your digestive tract functions. It starts with intake.

Erasmus, Udo. *Fats that Heal, Fats that Kill*. Burnaby, BC: Alive Books, 1993. For an overview of the statistics on altered fats/oils and disease, see pages 325 – 379.

Jensen, Bernard, and Anderson, Mark. *Empty Harvest: Understanding the Link Between Our Food, Our Immunity and Our Planet*. New York: Avery Publishing, 1973.

Nestle, Marion. *What to Eat*. New York: North Point Press, 2006.

Robbins, John. *Diet for a New America*. Tiburon, CA: HJ Kramer, 1987.

Suzuki, David. "Programmed to be Fat?" *The Nature of Things*. http://www.cbc.ca/natureofthings/episode/programmed-to-be-fat.html. For an overview of the current research on 'obesogens': This episode highlights the work of researchers Bruce Blumberg from the University of California at Irvine, Paula Baillie-Hamilton, a Visiting Fellow at Stirling University, Alison Holloway from McMaster University, Fred Vom Saal from the University of Missouri, Retha Newbold and Jerry Heindel from the U.S. National Institute for Environmental Health Sciences (NIEHS).

Week #4 – Find the Exercise that is Right for You

Brue, Suzanne. *The 8 Colors of Fitness*. Delray Beach, Florida: Oakledge Press, 2008.

Camhi, SM, et al. "Accelerometer-determined moderate intensity lifestyle activity and cardiometabolic health." *Preventative Medicine*, 2011 May;52(5):358-60.

Raichlen, Da, and Polk, JD. "Linking brains and brawn: exercise and the evolution of human neurobiology." *Proceedings of The Royal Society in Biological Sciences*, 7 January 2013 vol. 280 no. 1750, Published online November 2012.

Ratey, JJ, and Loehr, JE. "The positive impact of physical activity on cognition during adulthood: a review of the underlying mechanisms, evidence and recommendations." *Reviews in Neuroscience*, 2011;22(2):171-85.

Stern, SA, and Alberini, CM. "Mechanisms of memory enhancement." *Wiley Interdisciplinary Reviews/Systems Biology and Medicine*, 2013 Jan;5(1):37-53. doi: 10.1002/wsbm.1196. Epub 2012 Nov 13.

Week #5 – Fall in Love with Vegetables

Bowden, Jonny. *The 150 Healthiest Foods on Earth*. Beverly, MA: Fair Winds Press, 2007.

Heber, David. *What Color is Your Diet?* New York: HarperCollins, 2001.

Roberts, Susan. *The Instinct Diet: Use Your Five Food Instincts to Lose Weight and Keep it Off*. New York: Workman Publishing Co., December 2008.

Welch, AA, et al. "A higher alkaline dietary load is associated with greater indexes of skeletal muscle mass in women." *Osteoporosis International*, 2012 November 14.

Wolfe, David. *Eating for Beauty*. San Diego: Maul Brothers Publishing, March 2002.

Week #5 – Get in Tune With Your Hunger

Faulconbridge LF, and Hayes MR. "Regulation of energy balance and body weight by the brain: a distributed system prone to disruption." *The Psychiatric Clinics of North America*, 2011 Dec; 34(4):733-45. Epub 2011 Oct 11.

Rosenbaum, Michael, et al. "Leptin reverses weight loss–induced changes in regional neural activity responses to visual food stimuli." *The Journal of Clinical Investigation*, 2008;118(7):2583–2591.

UT Southwestern Medical Center. "Overproducing Leptin Receptors In Fat Cells May Be Key To Halting Weight Gain." *Science Daily*, 2 Dec. 2005. Web. 26 Dec. 2012.

Week #6 – Check Those Simple Carbs at the Door

Ebbeling, CB, et al. "Effects of Dietary Composition on Energy Expenditure During Weight-Loss Maintenance." *The Journal of the American Medical Association*, June 27, 2012, Vol 307, No. 24.

"Insulin and Glucagon." http://www.medbio.info/Horn/Time%203-4/homeostasis_2.htm

Week #6 – Identify Your 'Why of Overeating'

Adam, Tanja, and Epel, Elissa. "Stress, eating and the reward system." *Physiology & Behavior*, 91 (2007) 449–458.

Estroff Marano, Hara. "Stress and Eating." *Psychology Today,* online publication, November 21, 2003.

Heller, RF, and Heller, RF. *The Stress-Eating Cure: Lose Weight with the No-Willpower Solution to Stress-Hunger and Cravings.* Rodale Books, April 2010.

Somov, Pavel. *Eating the Moment: 141 Mindful Practices to Overcome Overeating One Meal at a Time.* Oakland, CA: New Harbinger Publications, October 2008.

Week #7 – Eat Good Fats, Get Rid of the Bad

Erasmus, Udo. *Fats that Heal, Fats that Kill.* Burnaby, BC: Alive Books, 1993. See pages 111, 326 – 327.

Gadgil, MD, et al. "The Effects of Carbohydrate, Unsaturated Fat, and Protein Intake on Measures of Insulin Sensitivity: Results from the OmniHeart Trial." *Diabetes Care*, 2012 Dec 5. [Epub ahead of print].

Galli, C, and Calder, PC. "Effects of fat and fatty acid intake on inflammatory and immune responses: a critical review." *Annals of Nutrition & Metabolism,* 2009; 55(1-3):123-39. Epub 2009 Sep 15.

Kalupahana, NS, Claycombe, KJ, and Moustaid-Moussa N. "(n-3) Fatty acids alleviate adipose tissue inflammation and insulin resistance: mechanistic insights." *Advances in Nutrition*, 2011 Jul;2(4):304-16. Epub 2011 Jun 28.

López-Alarcón M, et al. "Supplementation of n3 long-chain polyunsaturated fatty acid synergistically decreases insulin resistance with weight loss of obese prepubertal and pubertal children." *Archives of Medical Research*, 2011 Aug;42(6):502-8.

Noreen E, et al. "Effect of supplemental fish oil on resting metabolic rate and body composition in middle-aged adults." *Journal of the International Society of Sports Nutrition*, 2010, 7:31.

Schirmer, MA, and Phinney, SD. "Gamma-linolenate reduces weight regain in formerly obese humans." *The Journal of Nutrition*, 2007 Jun;137(6):1430-5.

Teegala, SM, Willett, WC, and Mozaffarian, D. "Consumption and health effects of trans fatty acids: a review." *Journal of AOAC International*, 2009 Sep-Oct;92(5):1250-7.

Vanderhaeghe, Lorna, and Karst, Karlene. *Healthy Fats for Life*. Canada: Wiley, 2004. [For an overview plus research references for GLA's role in both skin conditions and hormonal health.]

Wallace, SK and Mozaffarian, D. "Trans-fatty acids and nonlipid risk factors." *Current Artherosclerosis Reports*, 2009 Nov; 11(6):423-33.

An overview of the benefits of Omega 3 fats plus research references to support it can be found at http://www.umm.edu/altmed/articles/omega-3-000316.htm.

Week #7 – Take Charge of Your Emotions

Cahill, Larry. "Sex Influences of the Brain and Emotional Memory." Video available at www.youtube.com, published on April 9, 2012.

Grodzki, Lynn. "Approaching A Theory of Emotion: An Interview With Candace Pert, Ph.D." May 1995. http://www.primal-page.com/pert.htm

Institute of HeartMath. "Science of the Heart: Exploring the Role of the Heart in Human Performance: An Overview of Research Conducted by the Institute of HeartMath." Available for download at http://www.heartmath.org/research/science-of-the-heart/introduction.html.

Pert, Candace. *Molecules of Emotion: The Science Behind Mind-Body Medicine*. New York: Simon & Schuster, 1997.

Pert, CB, Dreher, HE, and Ruff, MR. "The psychosomatic network: foundations of mind-body medicine." *Alternative Therapies in Health and Medicine*, 1998, 4(4): 30 – 41.

Ratey, John. *A User's Guide to the Brain: Perception, Attention, and the Four Theaters of the Brain*. New York: Vintage Books, 2002.

Rein, Glen, Atkinson, Mike, and McCraty, Rolin. "The Physiological and Psychological Effects of Compassion and Anger." *Journal of Advancement in Medicine*, 1995; 8(2): 87 – 105.

Sternberg, Esther. *The Balance Within: The Science Connecting Health and Emotions*. New York: W.H. Freeman, 2001.

Week #8 – Get on Board with the 90/10 Rule

Kessler, David A. *The End of Overeating: Taking Control of the Insatiable North American Appetite*. Toronto: McClelland & Stewart Ltd., 2009

Ward, SJ, and Dykstra, LA. "The Role of CB1 Receptor Antagonism (Sr141716a) and CB1 Receptor Agonism (Cp-55940)," *Behavioural Pharmacology 16*, no 5 -6 (2005): 381 – 8

Week #8 – Nourish Your Soul

Bolte Taylor, Jill. *My Stroke of Insight: A Brain Scientist's Personal Journey*. New York: Penguin Group, June 2009.

Cunningham, Rosemary. "Fifty Ways to Nourish Your Soul." *Sprituiality & Health,* March – April, 2002. http://spiritualityhealth.com/articles/fifty-ways-nourish-your-soul

Fredrickson, Barbara. *Positivity: Groundbreaking Research Reveals How to Embrace the Hidden Strength of Positive Emotions, Overcome Negativity, and Thrive*. New York: Crown Publishing, 2009.

Heller, RF, and Heller, RF. *The Stress-Eating Cure: Lose Weight with the No-Willpower Solution to Stress-Hunger and Cravings.* Rodale Books, April 2010.

Week #9 – Rest and Relax to Lighten Up

Easton, John. "Lack of sleep alters hormones, metabolism." *The University of Chicago Chronicle,* Dec. 2, 1999, Vol. 19 No. 6.

Froy, O. "Metabolism and circadian rhythms--implications for obesity." *Endocrine Reviews,* 2010 Feb;31(1):1-24. Epub 2009 Oct 23.

Garfinkel, D., et al. "Efficacy and safety of prolonged-release melatonin in insomnia patients with diabetes: a randomized, double-blind, cross-over study." *Diabetes Metabolic Syndrome and Obesity,* 2011; 4: 307–313. Published online 2011 August 2.

Kobayashi, D., et al. "Association between weight gain, obesity, and sleep duration: a large-scale 3-year cohort study." *Sleep & Breathing,* 2012 Sep;16(3):829-33. Epub 2011 Sep 3.

Lucassen, EA, Rother, KI, and Cizza, G. "Interacting epidemics? Sleep curtailment, insulin resistance, and obesity." *Annals of the New York Academy of Sciences,* 2012 August; 1264(1): 110–134. Published online 2012 July 24.

Marino, Patrick. "Biological Rhythms as a Basis for Mood Disorders." Published online at http://www.personalityresearch.org/papers/marino.html

Nielsen, LS, Danielsen, KV, and Sorensen, TI. "Short sleep duration as a possible cause of obesity: critical analysis of the epidemiological evidence." *Obesity Reviews,* 2011 Feb; 12(2):78-92.

Patel, SR, et al. "Association between reduced sleep and weight gain in women." *American Journal of Epidemiology,* 2006 Nov 15;164(10):947-54. Epub 2006 Aug 16.

Patel SR, Hu FB. "Short sleep duration and weight gain: a systematic review." *Obesity (Silver Spring).* 2008; 16:643-53.

Spiegel K, Leproult R, Tasali E, Penev P, and Van Cauter E. "Sleep curtailment results in decreased leptin levels, elevated ghrelin levels and increased hunger and appetite." *Annals of Internal Medicine,* 2004;141(11):846-50.

Spiegel K, Leproult R, L'Hermite-Balériaux M, Copinschi G, Penev P and Van Cauter E. "Impact of sleep duration on the 24-hour leptin profile: relationships with sympatho-vagal balance, cortisol and TSH." *Journal of Clinical Endocrinology & Metabolism,* 2004; 89(11):5762-71.

Taheri, S, et al. "Short sleep duration is associated with reduced leptin, elevated ghrelin, and increased body mass index." *PLoS Medicine,* 2004 Dec;1(3):e62. Epub 2004 Dec 7.

The University of Chicago Medicine News Office. "Lack of deep sleep may increase risk of type 2 diabetes." December 31, 2007. http://www.uchospitals.edu/news/2007/20071231-diabetes.html

Vgontzas, Alexandro, et al. "Chronic Insomnia Is Associated with Nyctohemeral Activation of the Hypothalamic-Pituitary-Adrenal Axis: Clinical Implications." *JCEM,* 2001 August 86 (8): 3787.

Week #9 – Create a Healthy Relationship with Your Body

Blakeslee, Sandra, and Blakeslee, Matthew. *The Body Has a Mind of Its Own: How Body Maps in Your Brain Help You Do (Almost) Everything Better.* New York: Random House, 2007.

The written source for the visualization in this chapter has long been lost, although it remains entrenched in my memory. I originally heard it through my coach training with CTI, The Coaches Training Institute. I believe it was written by either Laura Whitworth or Karen Kimsey-House.

Week #10 – Take Control of Your Portions

Groves, Barry. "Do Calories Really Count?" Published online at http://www.second-opinions.co.uk/do-calories-really-count.html.

National Health and Welfare. Food Consumption Patterns Report. Ottawa: Bureau of Nutritional Sciences, 1977.

Thomas, Graeme. "Calorie Counting: Backasswards Diet Advice." Published online at http://graemethomasonline.com/calorie-counting-backasswards-diet-advice.

Statistics Canada. Canadian Community Health Survey, Nutrition, 2004. Available online at http://publications.gc.ca/collections/Collection/Statcan/82-620-M/82-620-MIE2006002.pdf?

Week #10 – Tackle Social Eating

Fox, Robin. "Food and Eating: An Anthropological Perspective." Online contribution to the Social Issues Research Center, www.sirc.org.

Week #11 – Learn to Navigate the Grocery Store

Corporate sponsors for the Canadian Foundation for Dietetic Research can be found at www.cfdr.ca. And for the Academy of Nutrition and Dietetics, their corporate sponsors can be found at www.eatright.org.

Hensel, Gerald. Global Brands. "The Illusion of Choice." Diagram published online at http://davaidavai.com/2012/04/25/global-brands-the-illusion-of-choice/.

Industry Report: Cereal Breakfast Foods. Published online at http://business.highbeam.com/industry-reports/food/cereal-breakfast-foods.

Kessler, David A. *The End of Overeating: Taking Control of the Insatiable North American Appetite.* Toronto: McClelland & Stewart Ltd., 2009

Nestle, Marion. *What to Eat.* New York: North Point Press, 2006.

http://everytable.wordpress.com/about/

Week #11 – Practice Mindful Eating

Giduck, SA, Threatte, RM, and Kare, MR. "Cephalic reflexes: their role in digestion and possible roles in absorption and metabolism." *Journal of Nutrition*, 1987 Jul;117(7):1191-6.

Higgs S, and Donohoe JE. "Focusing on food during lunch enhances lunch memory and decreases later snack intake." *Appetite*, 2011 Aug;57(1):202-6. Epub 2011 May 4.

LeBlanc J, and Cabanac M. "Cephalic postprandial thermogenesis in human subjects." *Physiology & Behavior*, 1989 Sep; 46(3): 479-82.

LeBlanc, J, Cabanac, M, and Samson, P. "Reduced postprandial heat production with gavage as compared with meal feeding in human subjects." *American Journal of Physiology*, 1984 Jan; 246(1 Pt 1):E95-101.

Morse, DR, et al. "Oral digestion of a complex-carbohydrate cereal: effects of stress and relaxation on physiological and salivary measures." *American Journal of Clinical Nutrition*, 1989 Jan;49(1):97-105.

Oldham-Cooper RE, et al. "Playing a computer game during lunch affects fullness, memory for lunch, and later snack intake." *American Journal of Clinical Nutrition*, 2011 Feb; 93(2):308-13. Epub 2010 Dec 8.

Sojcher R, Gould Fogerite S, and Perlman A. "Evidence and potential mechanisms for mindfulness practices and energy psychology for obesity and binge-eating disorder." *Explore (New York, NY)*, 2012 Sep; 8(5):271-6.

Wanden-Berghe RG, Sanz-Valero J, and Wanden-Berghe C. "The application of mindfulness to eating disorders treatment: a systematic review." *Eating Disorders*, 2011 Jan;19(1):34-48.

Week #12 – Consider Researched Supplements

Bakuradze T, et al. "Antioxidant-rich coffee reduces DNA damage, elevates glutathione status and contributes to weight control: results from the intervention study." *Molecular Nutrition & Food Research*, 2011;55:793–797.

Barrett ML, and Udani JK. "A proprietary alpha-amylase inhibitor from white bean (Phaseolus vulgaris): a review of clinical studies on weight loss and glycemic control." *Nutrition Journal*, 2011 Mar 17;10:24.

Basu, Arpita, et al. "Green Tea Supplementation Affects Body Weight, Lipids, and Lipid Peroxidation in Obese Subjects with Metabolic Syndrome." *Journal of American College of Nutrition*, 2010 29: 31-40.

Celleno L, et al. "A dietary supplement containing standardized Phaseolus vulgaris extract influences body composition of overweight men and women." *International Journal of Medical Science*, 2007 Jan 24;4(1):45-52.

Dellaibera B, Lemaire S, and Lafay S. "Svetol, green coffee extract, induces weight loss and increases the lean to fat mass ratio in volunteers with overweight problem."*Phytotherapie*, 2006; 4:194–197.

Downs BW, et al. "Bioefficacy of a novel calcium-potassium salt of (-)-hydroxycitric acid." *Mutation Research*, 2005 Nov 11;579(1-2):149-62. Epub 2005 Aug 1.

Gaullier JM, et al. "Conjugated linoleic acid supplementation for 1 year reduces body fat mass in healthy overweight humans." *American Journal of Clinical Nutrition*, 2004 Jun;79(6):1118-25.

Gaullier JM, et al. "Six months supplementation with conjugated linoleic acid induces regional-specific fat mass decreases in overweight and obese." *British Journal of Nutrition*, 2007 Mar;97(3):550-60.

Grove, Kimberly, and Lambert, Joshua. "Laboratory, Epidemiological, and Human Intervention Studies Show That Tea (Camellia sinensis) May Be Useful in the Prevention of Obesity." *Journal of Nutrition*, 2010 140: 446-453.

Krissansen GW. "Emerging health properties of whey proteins and their clinical implications." *Journal of the American College of Nutrition*, 26 (6): 713S–23S

Lau FC, Bagchi M, Sen C, Roy S, and Bagchi D. "Nutrigenomic analysis of diet-gene interactions of functional supplements for weight management."*Current Genomics*, 2008 Jun; 9(4):239-51.

Luhovyy BL, Akhavan T, and Anderson GH. "Whey Proteins in the Regulation of Food Intake and Satiety." *Journal of the American College of Nutrition*, December 2007 vol. 26 no. 6, 704S-712S

Maki KC, et al. "Green Tea Catechin Consumption Enhances Exercise-Induced Abdominal Fat Loss in Overweight and Obese Adults" *Journal of Nutrition*, February 1, 2009 139:264-270.

Market Research News. "Global market for weight loss worth US$586.3 billion by 2014." [Accessed November 18, 2011]. Available from: http://www.salisonline.org/market-research/global-market-for-weight-loss-worth-us586-3-billion-by-2014/

Markus CR, Jonkman LM, Lammers JH, Deutz NE, Messer MH, and Rigtering N. "Evening intake of alpha-lactalbumin increases plasma tryptophan availability and improves morning alertness and brain measures of attention." *American Journal of Clinical Nutrition*, 81:1026– 33, 2005.

Nagao T, Hase T, and Tokimitsu I. "A green tea extract high in catechins reduces body fat and cardiovascular risks in humans." *Obesity (Silver Spring)*, 2007;15:1473–83.

Nagao T, et al. "Ingestion of a tea rich in catechins leads to a reduction in body fat and malondialdehyde-modified LDL in men." *American Journal of Clinical Nutrition*, 2005; 81: 122–9.

Onakpoya IJ, Posadzki PP, Watson LK, Davies LA, and Ernst E. "The efficacy of long-term conjugated linoleic acid (CLA) supplementation on body composition in overweight and obese individuals: a systematic review and meta-analysis of randomized clinical trials." *European Journal of Nutrition*, 2012 Mar; 51(2):127-34. Epub 2011 Oct 12.

Preuss HG, et al. "An overview of the safety and efficacy of a novel, natural (-)-hydroxycitric acid extract (HCA-SX) for weight management." *Journal of Medicine*, 2004;35(1-6):33-48.

Risérus U, Berglund L, and Vessby B. "Conjugated linoleic acid (CLA) reduced abdominal adipose tissue in obese middle-aged men with signs of the metabolic syndrome: a randomised controlled trial." *International Journal of Obesity and Related Metabolic Disorders*, 2001 Aug;25(8):1129-35.

Thom E. "A randomized, double-blind, placebo-controlled trial of a new weight-reducing agent of natural origin." Journal of International Medical Research, 2000; 28:229–233.

Veldhorst MA, et al. "Effects of complete whey-protein breakfasts versus whey without GMP-breakfasts on energy intake and satiety." *Appetite*, 2009 Apr; 52(2):388-95. Epub 2008 Dec 3.

Wolfram S, Wang Y, and Thielecke F. "Anti-obesity effects of green tea: From bedside to bench." *Molecular Nutrition & Food Research*, 50 :176– 187,2006.

Vinson JA, Burnham BR, Nagendran MV. "Randomized, double-blind, placebo-controlled, linear dose, crossover study to evaluate the efficacy and safety of a green coffee bean extract in overweight subjects." *Diabetes, Metabolic Syndromes & Obesity*, 2012; 5:21-7. Epub 2012 Jan 18.

For a list of all sources of research on PGX, go to http://www.pgx.com/ca/en/articles/a5/the-science-of-pgx.

Environment

Christakis, Nicholas and Fowler, James. "The Spread of Obesity in a Large Social Network over 32 Years." *New England Journal of Medicine*, 2007; 357:370-379.

Heath, Chip, and Health, Dan. *Switch: How to Change Things When Change is Hard*. New York: Random House, 2010.

Fashion information re: 18th century England from www.americanrevolution.org

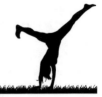

Acknowledgments

Writing this book was quite simply the longest running and most challenging project I have ever taken on and completed. It consumed my time and my mind for the last two years and despite loathing the idea of giving up my weekends, it was all I could do to complete it. Needless to say there have been many people along the way that have been instrumental in helping me to make it a physical reality.

Thanks to my book coach, Andrea Kennedy, who helped me solidify my ideas into a more cohesive picture. Andrea, you may not realize how critical your role was. I am not sure how I would have gotten through the mounds of inertia without your enthusiasm and belief in me as a writer. To my brother Winston, your generosity in sharing your time and insights has been invaluable. I needed you on my team. To Priscilla Beard, Lynn Spencer and Bruce Simpson for being not only exemplary clients, but also for allowing me to use your testimonials for the book cover. To my partner Barry, who despite not reading one word that I've written has provided unwavering belief in me, and my work. To my other brother Mark for his graphic talents and for making the cover better than it's original design. To my mom Betty for being so excited to see my book in print that she drove me to complete it. To my dearest friends Kristen Barrett and Joan Fast for their unwavering support, powerful questions and like-mindedness that have provided a sense of community in purpose. And to my son Sasha, for whom my love runs so deep that he more than anyone, has catalyzed me to be a better human being, so I could pass on something worthwhile.

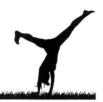

Index

Made in the USA
Charleston, SC
29 April 2013